Health, Communication and Multicultural Communities

Health, Communication and Multicultural Communities: Topics on Intercultural Communication for Healthcare Professionals

By

Carmen Valero-Garcés

CAMBRIDGE
SCHOLARS
PUBLISHING

Health, Communication and Multicultural Communities:
Topics on Intercultural Communication for Healthcare Professionals,
by Carmen Valero-Garcés

This book first published 2014

Cambridge Scholars Publishing

12 Back Chapman Street, Newcastle upon Tyne, NE6 2XX, UK

British Library Cataloguing in Publication Data
A catalogue record for this book is available from the British Library

ISBN (10): 1-4438-6027-1, ISBN (13): 978-1-4438-6027-7

Dedicated to my parents

TABLE OF CONTENTS

LIST OF FIGURES

LIST OF GRAPHS

LIST OF TABLES

PREFACE

Communication is an essential component of humans. The published literature also expresses belief in the essential role of communication in patient care. It shows that difficulties in the effective delivery of healthcare can arise from problems in communication between patient and provider rather than from any failing in the technical aspects of medical care and that improvement in provider-patient communication can have beneficial effects on health outcomes. It is within the healthcare sector that a greater number of multicultural encounters occur and where there is a great need for trained staff who can work to avert risk and save time and money while helping to support a right which the Bill of Human Rights recognizes as one to which all human beings should have access. Research related to effective communication in multicultural settings is also becoming increasingly abundant by way of publications, congresses, seminars and activities. Thanks to this increased activity, the topic is rapidly achieving greater recognition and is becoming much more interdisciplinary. This book provides an overview of current issues through a multi-faceted approach, situating the work of potential healthcare professionals and intercultural intermediaries in the broader context of public service providers and practitioners. It also intends to help fill the vacuum in the market of educational materials focused on different language pairs or on those minority languages in which communication is difficult without some sort of third party link. However, this book could not have become a reality without the help of many professionals.

My first thanks go to all those who helped me in this work over the years, especially medical staff, foreign patients, colleagues and students of the postgraduate program in Intercultural Communication, Public Service Interpreting and Translation at the University of Alcalá (Madrid), Spain, who opened up several research paths and contributed with information, experience and data. I have fond memories and great respect for doctors and medical staff of hospitals and healthcare centers in the central area of Spain. Their dedication and respect towards the many foreign patients they had to attend on an everyday basis; often inspiring some of the topics found in this book. The basic research for the original versions of some of the articles in this volume would not have been possible without the contribution of migrant patients. Finally, the production would not have been possible if were it not for my many years of research on the healthcare setting, the consolidation of the FITISPos group, the contributions of colleagues, the work and effort of students and future public service translators and my own experience coordinating and teaching the Training and Research Program in Public Service Interpreting and Translation at the University of Alcalá, Madrid, Spain as well as at the different associations and organizations in Spain, whose collaboration has been essential to seeing this project to its end. I would like to acknowledge all the Masters and PhD candidates we have worked with over the years, who have contributed to my thinking about the most effective approaches to conducting interdisciplinary research and also lead me and the group FITISPos to identify the need for this book and other publications. I would like to give my most profound thanks to all of them, and especially to Cristina Balaban, Ashley Krewatch and Marianna Musacchio, who contributed with their investigations to develop some of the chapters of this book. I would also like to recognize the diligent work of Amy Tobin and Brian Assaf, who assisted with the translations, revision and copyediting of the book.

I hope that all of the efforts of everybody involved in this book are recognized and followed upon by the readers of these pages. This book in your hands is further proof that we are moving toward multilingual and multicultural societies where languages and cultures are weaving unimaginable webs and where cooperation and interdisciplinary knowledge are more needed than ever before. Interest is growing in many different academic, institutional, professional, and social circles in which we take part. This interest also calls attention to past errors, current needs and the future projects that will be required to solve the difficulties we encounter along the long road toward the consolidation of multilingual communities. Knowledge, research, training, collaboration, and practice are some of the keys to achieving this goal. I truly believe and hope that this book will be helpful in these areas and will be another step towards the successful development of joint actions in the domain of communication in multicultural settings, a field important to those involved in ensuring access to healthcare.

Carmen Valero-Garcés
Alcalá de Henares, May 2014

List of Transcription Symbols

Conventions of Transcription and symbols used :

[…] = Pause or silence
(¿????) = Poor acoustics and what the speaker said was not transcribed
} = overlap
D = Doctor
P = Patient
N= Nurse

LIST OF ABBREVIATIONS

ASL (American Sign Language)
AUSIT (Australian Institute of Interpreters and Translators Incorporated)
CCHCP (Cross Cultural Health Care Program)
CHIA (California Healthcare Interpreters Association)
EFSIL (European Forum of Sign Language Interpreters)
ESSP (English Speaking Survey Participants)
FILSE (Federación Española de Interpretes de Lengua de Signos).
FITISPos (Formación e Investigación en Traducción e Interpretación en los Servicios Públicos/Training and Research in Public Service Translation and Interpreting) group in Spain
IMIA (International Medical Interpreters Association)
IoL (Institute of Linguists, United Kingdom)
LEP (Limited English Proficiency)
L1 (First Language)
L2 (Second Language)
MMIA (Massachusetts Medical Interpreters Association)
NAATI (National Accreditation Authority for Translators and Interpreters, Australia)
NCIHC (National Council of Interpreting in Health Care, USA)
NRPSI (National Register of Public Service Interpreters, UK)
NSSP (Non-Spanish speaking Patients)
PSIT (Public Service Interpreting and Translation)
RID (Registry of Interpreters for the Deaf, EE UU and Canada)
STK (Small Talk)
SL (Source Language)
ST (Source Text)
TT (Target Text)

INTRODUCTION

PATIENT - DOCTOR COMMUNICATION

Communicating in multicultural settings is a field of central interest to those involved in ensuring access to healthcare. Ever increasing migration requires access to essential legal, medical and social services. This book provides an overview of current issues through a multi-faceted approach, situating the work of potential healthcare professionals and intercultural intermediaries in the broader context of public service providers and practitioners.

Extensive research has shown that no matter how knowledgeable the physician might be, if he or she is unable to open an effective channel of communication with the patient, then he or she will likely be of little help to that patient. Asnani (2009: 357- 361) in her article “Patient - physician communication” concludes that, despite this and the fact that a patient-physician consultation is the most widely performed 'procedure' in a physician's professional lifetime, effective communication with the patient has been found to be sadly lacking. If we add the element of 'multilingual and multicultural' to this communication, the situation worsens. This proposal seeks to offer some solutions.

Research related to effective communication in multicultural settings is becoming increasingly abundant by way of publications, congresses, seminars and activities. Thanks to this increased activity, the topic is rapidly achieving greater recognition and is becoming much more interdisciplinary. Faced with the need to respond to the new challenges raised by immigration and the advance towards multicultural societies that has taken place in the last few decades, it has become evident that both healthcare providers and patients must improve their communication in order to avoid misunderstandings and the negative consequences there of. When language and / or culture is an obstacle, new needs and solutions must be developed: Utilizing a third person who knows the languages and cultures involved and thereby can act as a link between provider and patient; training bilinguals to become professional communicators (interpreters, mediators, translators); making resources available in different languages (brochures, dictionaries, etc.); training service providers to work in multicultural settings; building awareness around the sociocultural differences between communities and how said differences influence communication and daily life; learning how to work with interpreters and / or mediators to name but a few.

Nevertheless, there is scarcely any educational material on the market focused on different language pairs or on those minority languages in which communication is difficult without some sort of third party link. Nor are there specific materials geared at helping service providers or medical staff to understand their customers or patients in the public administration, hospitals, health clinics or schools.

Communication is an important component of patient care. Traditionally, communication in medical school curricula has not existed at all or has been scantily and informally incorporated as part of rounds and faculty feedback. The reliability and consistency of this teaching method leave gaps, which currently receive increased attention from medical schools and accreditation organizations. With the move towards multilingual and multicultural societies, there is also an increased interest in researching patient-doctor communication and recognizing the need to teach and measure this specific clinical skill.

The published literature also expresses belief in the essential role of communication. It shows that difficulties in the effective delivery of health care can arise from problems in communication between patient and provider rather than from any failing in the technical aspects of medical care and that improvement in provider-patient communication can have beneficial effects on health outcomes.

Patient – Physician relationship is also changing. Historically in medicine, there was a paternalistic approach to deciding what should be done for a patient: the physician knew best and the patient accepted the recommendation without question. This era is changing and patients are advising to ask questions and to be informed and to have access to quality information. Patient satisfaction with their care, rests heavily on how successfully this transition is accomplished. A great number of multicultural encounters take place within the healthcare setting and thus, there is a great need for resources such as trained staff who can work to avert risk, and – as research shows- to save time and money.

Most of the working materials and examples are taken from authentic materials. Many of these come from the English-Spanish language pair, since this is a language pair with a dual profile. In the case of English, it is undoubtedly the *lingua franca* in the professional arena, but it is also the linking language in encounters between the dominant and minority communities in immigration settings (e.g between Spanish and Swahili).

In the case of Spanish, it is the third most spoken language in the word, but it is also the minority language spoken among many migrants in a large number of EU countries as well as in the USA, where it represents the dominant minority. In addition, Spain is the EU country which has had the most migration in the last few decades and where the advances towards a multicultural society mean that strategies must be developed to cope with the challenges posed by the new situation.

It is within the healthcare sector that a greater number of multicultural encounters occur and where there is a great need for trained staff who can work to avert risk and save time and money while helping to support a right which the Bill of Human Rights recognizes as one to which all human beings should have access. Thus, even though Spanish and English are used as examples, a lot of the information presented in the book can be extrapolated to other language pairs.

Following there is a chapter breakdown of the contents. Each chapter includes examples and activities that can either be used for self-study or as a textbook to be used in class.

Chapter 1 - Health, Communication and the - Migrant Population. - illustrates certain realities of the communication that takes place between the migrant community and those working in the healthcare sector, especially in those cases where there is no shared language or culture. To begin, I will attempt to define this communication and the agents involved.

Chapter 2 - Communicating in Multilingual Settings. - is devoted to an analysis of the elements which play a role in the chain of linguistic communication, the different types of encounters that occur in medical consults and the problems that arise.

Chapter 3 - Changes in the Healthcare Setting. Perceptions from the Field about the Use of the Language - provides a description of the current state and evolution of health care services in a specific country evolving into multicultural societies where intercultural communication is a necessity.

Chapter 4 - English as a *Lingua Franca*. A Resource for Communication in Multilingual Medical Appointments - is an extension of Chapter 3 insomuch as it focuses on the use of the English language as a bridge to communicating with non-Spanish-speaking patients in the healthcare clinics and institutions of Spain.

Chapter 5 - Topics: Informed Consent and the Quality of Communication – presents a specific case of communication in doctor-patient consultations: the use of the informed consent with respect to doctor / non-native patient encounters illustrated with questions that arise such as: What happens when the patient does not "understand" the text? Or, how can one exercise their right to understand and be understood?

Chapter 6 - Negotiation of Meaning in Medical Consultations - focus on providing an analysis of the medical consultation and how meaning is negotiated in this institutional context using a very specific but extremely relevant type of discourse known as *small talk*.

Chapter 7 - Rapport Management Strategies in Intercultural Medical Encounters - might be considered an extension of the study presented in the previous chapter on the use of language in the medical encounter in two types of interactions: health care professional – Spanish patient, and health care professional – foreign patient.

Chapter 8 - Healthcare Providers and Interpreters Working as a Professional Team - help to fill a void which has been the subject of much discussion and the focus of this book: healthcare professional- and communication experts (interpreters and translators) in multilingual settings.

The book is not oriented towards one population in particular, but rather it is directed towards multiple groups, mainly to students of the health sciences and medical staff interested in communicating with the migrants and visitors or those who have to work in multicultural settings.

More specifically, the book is addressed at:

1. Future professionals in the healthcare and medical setting. The goal is to provide them with the theoretical knowledge, skills, competence and tools necessary to communicate effectively in multilingual / multicultural settings.
2. Future linguistic mediators (translating and interpreting professionals). The goal is to provide them with the theoretical knowledge, skills, competence and tools necessary to act as linguistic, communicative and cultural liaisons in the healthcare setting, so they can serve as a bridge between staff and clients who do not know or speak the contact language well.
3. Healthcare and medical professionals who, due to various circumstances, work in a multilingual / multicultural setting and need to strengthen their knowledge in order to communicate effectively.

In a broader sense, the book is directed at:

1. People who have experience as linguistic mediators either through oral or written communication, but who have not received any type of formal instruction.

2. People with experience in translating and interpreting who want to specialize in healthcare.
3. Trainers or developers of educational programs.
4. Those individuals who, for one reason or another, work in multilingual/multicultural settings and need to strengthen their knowledge in order to communicate effectively.

It is not a theoretical book nor is it rule-based by any means. It is a handbook oriented towards reflection and practice born from years of experience training mediators, interpreters and translators working in minority languages within multicultural settings. It can be used for self-study and independent learning, but will also be extremely useful to teachers and trainers of future doctors and medical staff who seek materials or readings for their classes. Furthermore, it will be an excellent resource for mediators, interpreters and translators who want to learn more about communication in healthcare setting.

Bibliographic references

Asnani, MR. "Patient-physician communication". *West Indian Med J.* 2009, Sep; 58 (4), 357-61.

CHAPTER ONE

HEALTH, COMMUNICATION AND THE MIGRANT POPULATION

Key Points

- The migrant population in healthcare settings
- The communication chain
- The migrant community and the Ulysses Syndrome
- Communicative competence and its importance in the therapeutic process

Key Readings

Achotegui, J. (2002). *La Depresión en los Inmigrantes: Una Perspectiva Transcultural*. Barcelona: Ediciones Mayo, S.A.

Clyne, M. (1994). *Inter-cultural Communication at Work: Cultural Values in Discourse*. Cambridge: Cambridge University Press.

Gumperz, J. (1982). *Discourse Strategies*. Cambridge: Cambridge University Press.

Poyatos, F. (1993). *Paralanguage: A Linguistic and Interdisciplinary Approach to Interactive Speech and Sounds.* Amsterdam/Philadelphia: John Benjamins.

1.1 Introduction. The migrant population and communication in healthcare settings

The primary goal of this chapter is to illustrate certain realities of the communication that takes place between the migrant community and those working in the healthcare sector, especially in those cases where there is no language or culture in common. To begin, I will attempt to define this communication and the agents involved; I will then contextualize the phenomenon of migration as it affects healthcare, given the fact that this is one of the most important sectors in countries such as Spain. I will be using Spain as an example and will be analyzing its characteristics and needs. Further along I will discuss another key agent in this communication: the healthcare worker. I will likewise analyze his or her characteristics and the difficulties he or she faces, paying special attention to the two groups which provide care to the greatest volume of migrants and visitors; primary care providers and nursing staff. This will lead us into a brief discussion of transcultural medicine and nursing and I will conclude by providing some key recommendations for the future in light of the challenges posed by the 21st century.

1.2 Communicating with the migrant community

The characteristics of the migrant patients that typically go to healthcare clinics and hospitals are without a doubt expressed in the profile which Carballo (2006) sets out and which is illustrated in the table below (Box 1.1.):

Box 1.1.

Some Characteristics of the Migrant Population	
-	Alienation and chronic sadness
-	A more stressful experience depending on gender
-	Rarely with family
-	Economic insecurity
-	Legal insecurity
-	Difficulties with the language
-	Difficulties with the culture
-	Difficulties with the social environment
-	Social and political-legal rejection

However, as Martincano (2003) reminds us, we are prevented from assigning any one homogeneous classification to all migrants given the diversity in life cycles. In other words, as people migrate to a country, they modify, acquire and adopt changes to their personal and social patterns of behavior, including those which impact their health (reproductive health, mental health, contagious diseases, occupational health…). Nevertheless, these people bring with them languages and cultures that are far-removed from the majority culture. This will inevitably lead to friction and will require both parties to make an effort to get along.

Based on this situation, it stands to reason that difficulties will also arise in the doctor-patient relationship, which may prevent the migrant patient from (fully) accessing the healthcare system for different reasons: a limited to total lack of knowledge of the official language, different opinions regarding health, illness or pain, lack of knowledge about how the country's healthcare system operates or about healthcare policy.

More than a decade ago Talero Martín (1997) described the main barriers that a patient comes up against when trying to access health care in Spain. These barriers can be classified into three groups: those stemming from the health care system, those related to the patient himself and those which are dependent on the health care professional. They are illustrated below in Box 1.2.:

Box 1.2.

Barriers in the Health Care Process		
Stemming from System	***Dependent on healthcare professional***	***Related to patient***
- Inadequate accessibility - Excessive wait time - Excessive demand/too little time for appointment - Noise and interruptions - Excessive beaurocracy	- Dysfunctional personality for clinic - Professional in charge of evaluation, or consult - Projects too much onto patient - Exhibits excessive control - Shows low empathy - Emotional interference - Issues related with the job itself - Problems in professional's personal life - Lack of training in communication skills - Lack of training in mental health issues - Social interference	- Physical problems: aphasia, hearing loss… - Emotions at breaking point: anxiety, aggressiveness… - Abnormal personalities: overly-dependant, obsessive - Somatoform disorders - Non-compliant patients - Frequency of visits - Language barriers - Social interference: Sociocultural distance.

Based on Martín Talero's profile, we can conclude that the healthcare system is complicated, extremely bureaucratic and totally inaccessible for anyone unfamiliar with how it operates in Spain (i.e. prescheduled appointments, long lines, infinite service windows, etc.) or who do not speak the official language.

According to Martincano (2003), the situation in terms of accessing the health care system underwent very little change in the first decade of the 21st century. This is illustrated below in Box 1.3.:

Box 1.3.

Issues with Migrant Access to the National Healthcare System (Spanish acronym - SNS)
- Active abandonment - Lack of knowledge - Bureaucratic complexity - Obstacles posed by local authorities - Difficulties with language - Cultural and religious questions - Social and labor difficulties

An important factor that can affect the quality of healthcare is the degree of empathy and how it is expressed or what we might call "social interference on the part of the professional". This social interference can stir up a variety of emotions, as shown in Box 1.4.:

Box 1.4.

Social Interference from Professional		
Ethnocentrism	Prejudice	Agression
Xenophobia	Stereotypes	Abusive behavior
Segregation	Discrimination	Exclusion
Racism	Hate	Social Exclusion
New racism	Rejection	Legal Exclusion
Ethnosensitivity	Information Have-nots	Exclusion from
	Recognize and appreciate differences	information

These emotions tend to come to the surface especially when a medical provider's work with the patient stirs up unresolved feelings of oppression and prejudice within him. This is due to the phenomenon of transference and countertransference that occurs within the doctor-patient relationship.

The outcome will depend on the direction of these emotions and the provider's attitudes towards the migrant patient. This is explained in more detail in the following chart (Figure 1.1) (Martincano 2003):

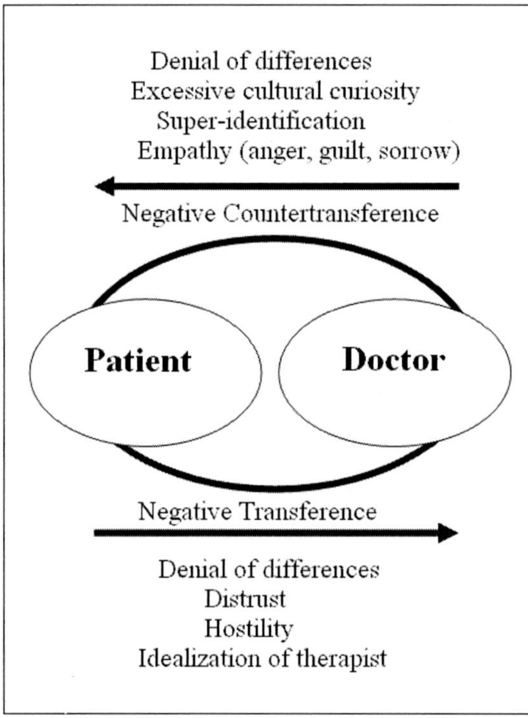

Figure 1.1: Providers' attitudes

The outcome also has to do with the tendency to apply the traditional model of western medicine. This model is characterized by medical paternalism and the doctor's role as part of a professional and social group which assumes the responsibility for healthcare. It is rooted in ethnocentrism and not in cultural relativism. Were the latter applied, it would allow for more flexibility and curiosity, as well as the desire to recognize and explore the intercultural components of the patient's feelings, show respect for other cultures and take a more sensitive approach to other customs.

1.3 The Ulysses Syndrome

Mental health of the migrant patient is also a key element in the provision of primary care, owing to the enormous influence that migration can have on the mental health of a patient. López Izquierdo, Martín del Barco and Álvarez (2007: 3 (5): 259-266) believe there are a number of factors that can make the migrant's experience so stressful: leaving behind family and one's homeland, the break with one's culture and customs, having to face a new society, experiencing difficult situations (unemployment, marginalization, discrimination), or the need to adapt to changes that lead to an imbalance between the demands of one's environment and one's ability to meet these demands and changes to which he/she is subjected.

This phenomenon is known as migratory grief and it involves the development of certain defense mechanisms that are expressed as: denial, projection (rejection, xenophobia), idealization and rationalization. When these mechanisms fail, the migrant may begin to suffer from depression and anxiety disorders, and then, he/she may develop the Immigrant Syndrome with Chronic and Multiple Stress, or Ulysses Syndrome (Achotegui 2002).

Described for the first time in 2002 by psychiatrist Joseba Achotegui from the Universitat de Barcelona, the Ulysses Syndrome refers to a set of symptoms experienced by people who leave their countries of origin to settle in an unknown land. The name of the syndrome is taken from the legendary Greek king of Ithaca depicted in Homer's poem, the Odyssey. This epic tale describes Ulysses' 10 years of struggles as he tries to return home after the war and claim his rightful place as the king of Ithaca.

The Ulysses Syndrome potentially affects anyone who migrates to a new country and faces the chronic stress that typically comes with adaptation to a different culture. It includes both physical and psychological symptoms, such as those of depression and anxiety, as well as somatic and dissociative symptoms ranging from headaches to clinical depression.

Martincano (2001) defines this as a specific disease linked to the intense nature of the chronic stress brought on by solitude, the battle for survival, frustration and the sense of failure felt by migrants. It is characterized by the presence of countless external stress factors of extreme intensity. This syndrome can be chronic, lasting for months or years. Figure 1.2 shows a summary of the stress factors involved in the psychopathological development of the migrant patient:

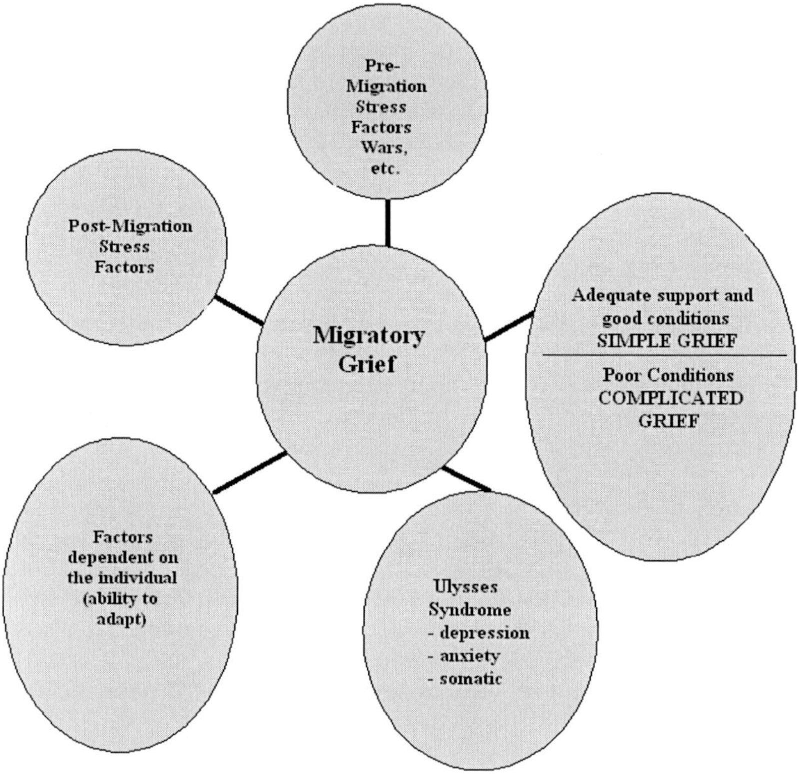

Figure 1.2: Stress factors

Following Achotegui (2002), the main stressors which cause this syndrome are:

1) Loneliness, especially present when the newcomer has left children and spouse behind. The overwhelming majority of migrants quickly realize how painful that first stage in the process of integration to a new country is, a process that starts with mourning all they have left behind.
2) Sense of despair and failure. Very often the migrant invests everything he or she had only to find that they cannot find the conditions to make even a decent living or fulfill their professional goals in the new country.

3) Survival struggles. Instead of fulfilling the dream of improved quality of life and being able to save enough money to send home or to provide a "better future" to their offspring, migrants often find themselves hardly making ends meet. People suffering from Ulysses Syndrome experience fear because of the uncertain future, and the struggle to survive overshadows all other priorities.
4) The risks endured in the process of migrating and settling down.

As for its treatment, recognizing the advances of the International Psychiatric research in demonstrating varying degrees of efficacy for improving and managing most advanced mental disorders through either psychotherapy (including talk therapy) and the use of medication (antidepressant, tranquilizers, stimulants, and a wide range of anti-psychotics), Diaz et al (2013) criticize the treatment frequently given for the Ulysses syndrome, which consists of simply increasing the prescription dose of this sort of medication. The example that follows illustrates their comments:

Box 1.5.

The case of Teresa, a migrant girl from Central America, who is one of many of newly arrived migrants experiencing the Ulysses Syndrome, including sadness, migraines, fatigue and bone pains. Teresa was seen by her general and primary physician who without providing her with any form of health education in Spanish, her native language (e.g., brochure, flyer, booklet or basic information), proceeded to prescribe her Prozac, a medication used by adults for the treatment of major depressive disorder, panic disorder, obsessive-compulsive disorder, and treatment-resistant depression. The medication did not alleviate Teresa's symptoms of sadness (i.e., homesickness). Rather, it worsened the initial condition and induced undesirable side effects, including lack of coordination, increased anxiety, impulsive and dangerous behavior, and thoughts about suicide. Her case illustrates how physicians often over prescribe medication, and minimize the evidence of dependency and adverse secondary drug reactions, especially to migrants of different cultural backgrounds experiencing extreme levels of stress. (Diaz et al. *The Ulysses Syndrome: Migrants with Chronic and Multiple Stress Symptoms and the Role of Indigenous Linguistically and Culturally Competent Community Health Workers*. 2013:4)

According to these authors, “the extensive therapeutic use of stimulants and a large number of psychoactive drugs in the cases of the many migrants with chronic and multiple stress syndrome, represents not only the ethnocentric medical approach in the west as the only valid and scientifically objective approach, but also a means of unjust social control of this population”. As globalization continues to permeate all social layers, this point of view is being increasingly supported by researchers and practitioners. As Diaz et al state, the diagnosis of depression is an easy way out and fits into a particular Western medical and cultural model, which reduces the psycho-social problem of an individual who in the diagnosis, is abstracted from a socioeconomic content and then held solely responsible for his / her mental well being.

Going against this tendency and in line with Achotegui’s studies, they propose a sociocultural approach rooted in a well designed and a well monitored community-based program as a means to identify and help migrants experiencing the Ulysses Syndrome.

To summarize, the inability to communicate due to the language barrier is a factor that must be taken into account, given that it can lead to different kinds of health-related complications for the migrant patient that can manifest as the condition known as Ulysses syndrome. This is a condition suffered by those who miss their homes, family and culture, which they have been forced to leave behind due to professional or personal circumstances, and who are unable to find a place in society. This inability to find one’s place in society is very much linked to the inability to communicate within one’s surroundings due to language.

1.4 Communicative competence beyond the words

Migration is, thus, an important life event which is influenced by many factors and which can have diverse consequences, one of which is without a doubt the consequence on health. It is a change which typically prompts other important life events (loss of or being uprooted from one’s family, language, customs, land, religion, culture, physical safety, economic changes, social activities, type of work, etc.) which can all affect the person’s health. As a consequence, doctor’s offices – especially in the primary care setting – are full of migrant patients with health problems who bring with them different practices and beliefs around health, the way a person becomes sick or is cured of illness.

These new patients therefore create new needs which must then be met. The first step must be achieving awareness of this new reality. My focus will be on one of the many elements of this reality: communication in medical consultations. I will discuss two kinds of communication which are practically inseparable: verbal and non-verbal communication and I will attempt to define terms such as: language, paralanguage, kinesics, proxemics, time and space, symbols and images, gaze and body contact.

I will begin by discussing verbal communication, which is one of the principal barriers in the doctor-patient relationship but also a barrier to the patient's right to understand and be understood. This is a right which is recognized on both an international level (Human Rights Declaration) as well as nationally.

Box 1.6.

Spain. Patient's right to understand and be understood Spanish Constitution, Organic Law *8/2000, of the 22 of December, Reform of the Organic Law 4/2000, of the 11 of January, regarding rights and freedoms of foreigners in Spain and their Social Integration. Or the current Health Care Law* (Law 41/2002).

Language is also linked to a series of codes which vary between different languages and which can lead to misunderstandings, skewed or ambiguous information. Frequently, one attempts to substitute these codes for other paralinguistic elements such as gestures or drawings. This is not simply a trivial observation but is one which is supported by numerous studies (Gumperz 1985, Poyatos 1994, Clyne 1994, Scollon and Scollon 1995).

Language cannot be separated out from culture, and there are numerous gaps in communication when there is no language in common. Some of these gaps are due to the reasons explained in the chart that follows:

Box 1.7.

Gaps in communication due to: Lack of vocabulary, lack of concepts, too wordy, scarcity of information, use of very formal language, unexpected greetings or topics that come up which deviate from appointment's typical structure, different ways of informing someone that they are sick, taboos or differences when considering what is or is not a disease (stress or anxiety).

Additionally, there are extralinguistic elements which accompany the message (paralanguage). These elements differ from culture to culture and affect communication. The chart below shows some of these paralinguistic elements.

Box 1.8.

Paralanguage elements affecting communication: Tone, vocal intensity, entonation and fluidity of language, as well as moments of silence and how long these silences last.

A doctor who feels uncomfortable with silence and barely allows for it might be intimidating to a patient – especially if the patient is Asian – for whom silence represents a sign of courtesy and not an invitation for the other to speak.

Box 1.9.

Gestures are not universal either, nor are the movements we make with certain parts of our body (kinesics), including our faces, the so-called mirror to the soul. Thus, facial expressions (smiles, grimaces), visual conduct (blinking, direction, scope and duration of gaze), or how we choose to beautify our faces (cosmetics, color, hair length, piercings) will have different meaning for different cultures.

Box 1.10.

Staring into another person's **eyes**, speaking in a loud **voice**, interrupting the speaker to **say** something, showing agreement by moving your **head** or smiling, keeping hands under the table or reaching out one's hand as a gesture to help are all gestures which can be used and interpreted in different ways.

Thus, if a patient avoids looking the doctor in the eyes when responding or when the doctor speaks to him, this does not necessarily signify a lack of honesty or interest. The value system of many Asian countries is different compared to that of Western cultures. Therefore, looking into the eyes of a superior is disrespectful and in those cultures, men are considered superior to women, as are fathers to their sons, teachers to students, doctors to nurses and so on and so forth. In the Muslim culture, among other differences which exist, if a man and woman look into each other's eyes it is considered to be an invitation of a sexual nature while two men holding hands in the street is not viewed as a sign of homosexuality.

Style of **dress** and the intended meaning also varies from one culture to another.

For example, removing one's hat upon entering the doctor's office is not a universal sign of respect. Furthermore, what can be said about symbols and images? These can be interpreted differently by different cultures. For someone from Asia an owl signifies insanity, the snake is reminiscent of poison, a cow is sacred, a dog is despised, white is the color of mourning and a black cat is a symbol of bad luck. As research has shown (Hablamos Juntos project), even those symbols which we deem to be universal in the medical setting (emergency signs, lab, x-ray, hospital…) are not always understood by all patients. Being aware of these elements will avoid misunderstandings on both sides.

Box 1.11.

The use of **personal space** (proxemics) is also different from one culture to another.

Each culture has its own rules. These rules are rarely written down nor are they taught when learning the language but they are nonetheless observed by all members of the group. We do not maintain the same distance when we are talking to Spaniards as we do when talking to the British or Americans or to Moroccans or people from China. Neither touch nor physical contact is viewed in the same way: while men in the Muslim world might walk hand in hand, those from Japan rarely touch one another. Thus, while for some, physical contact or keeping only a slight distance may show approval, empathy, protection, gentleness, or trust, for others this can seem almost aggressive. And the same is true for the doctor, who could start to exhibit a kind of rejection towards the patient if the patient gets too close, leans over the desk, or is overly demonstrative when saying hello or goodbye.

Box 1.12.

The value of **time**, the concept of time as linear or circular, arriving to an appointment late or the time one dedicates to initial greetings and niceties is also different.

Eastern European Catholics greet one another with a handshake using the right hand, along with a hug and two kisses on each cheek. The Arab Muslims, Jewish and Russians greet one another with a handshake, a hug, and polite questions about one's prosperity, well-being, family, weather, trip or about the place one comes from or lives, and other topics of that nature. In some cultures (e.g. Polynesian cultures) this initial interaction can last several minutes before the real conversation begins. The Russians respond to these questions carefully, since it would be considered rude to supply a short answer. When confronted with such a response, the doctor might become impatient and cut the person off, which would be insulting to the patient, as we have affirmed in some cases. (Taibi & Valero 2004).

1.5 The non-verbal code

All of the above is part of communication but all are nonverbal elements or, as Neuliep (2009) defines it, "the messages that people send to each other that do not contain words. He goes on to add that "this includes messages sent via body motions, vocal qualities, the use of time, space, artifacts, dress, and even smell", and dedicates a chapter to the non-verbal code. A brief explanation of the elements included in the non-verbal code follows:

Box 1.13.

The Non-verbal code (Neuliep): Kinesics, Paralanguage, Proxemics, Haptics and Olfactics

a) Communication with the body, called kinesics, consists of gestures, hand and arm movements, leg movements, facial expressions, eye gaze and blinking, and stance or posture.
b) Paralanguage, or the use of the voice, refers to vocal characteristics such as volume, pitch, rate, etc. Paralanguage can be divided into two broad categories, including voice qualities, and vocalizations. Paralinguistic voice qualities include such things as pitch, rhythm, tempo, articulation, and resonance of the voice. Paralinguistic vocalizations include laughing, crying, sighing, belching, swallowing, clearing of the throat, snoring, etc. Other paralinguistic vocalizations include intensity and non-fluencies such as "um," "ah," and "uh." Silence is also considered within the domain of paralanguage.

c) By studying space, or proxemics, we can learn how people express intimacy and power. Proxemics refers to the perception and use of space, including territoriality and personal space. Territoriality refers to physical geographical space and personal space refers to perceptual or psychological space; sometimes thought of as the "bubble" of space that humans carry with them during their day to day activities.
d) Haptics, or tactile communication refers to the use of touch, which may be the most primitive form of communication. Haptic communication varies widely across cultures, and the amount and kind of touch varies with the age, sex, situation and relationship of the people involved.
e) Through smell, called olfactics, a person's ethnicity, social class, and status are communicated.

Box 1.14.

The difference between verbal and nonverbal communication:
"Verbal communication represents the literal content of a message whereas the nonverbal component communicates the style or 'how' the message is to be interpreted. Hence, the nonverbal code often *complements, accents, substitutes, repeats* or even *contradicts* the verbal message" (Neuliep, 2009).

The work of Poyatos (1976, 1993), Candlin and Candlin (2003) or Helman (1990) on this topic offers a more complete vision on nonverbal communications that is also worth exploring.

The information provided by Neuliep applies to intercultural communication in healthcare settings because patients tend to orally describe how they are feeling during medical visits, accompanied by nonverbal gestures and other types of body language. The messages sent by patients, both verbally and nonverbally, are important for the healthcare specialists to comprehend in order for them to make serious decisions regarding the patient's course of action. The ability to take in both types of messages is not always easy, even in situations where both doctor and patient share the same mother tongue.

However, when doctor and patient do not share the same mother tongue, the situation becomes more complicated. In that case, one must consider the possibility that body language is not always universal. In fact, even in a monolingual situation where the patient is able to and chooses to speak in the doctor's native language, the body language may correspond to the patient's first language (L1), rather than crossing over to the second language (L2) that is being spoken. Thus Kellerman and Van Hoof (2003) found that Spanish speaking patients when using their L2 (English), their gestures did not conform to the patterns observed for the American and British speakers of English in the study. The authors concluded that although speaking their L2 fluently, the Spanish participants' gestures revealed that they had 'transferred' their L1 pattern of gesture use (Kellerman, van Hoof, 2003 as cited in McCafferty & Stam 2008).

1.6 Moving towards transcultural communication in healthcare

All the elements that we have discussed up until this point might be considered obvious to specialists in discourse analysis or language professionals. However, this is not always the case for professionals in other fields, who might not be aware of the importance of these elements or who have not received any training on communication techniques or who do not realize how important language is, all of which can be destructive to the medical consult.

Some problems related to language and culture that occur in the doctor-patient relationship are summarized by López Izquierdo et al (2007) as follows:

- Difficulty defining the reason for the consult
- Loss of nuances during communication
- Doctor doubts patient compliance
- Doctor doubts his own approach to the problem
- Patient shows lack of trust towards anyone who does not know his language
- More time is required for consult
- Difficulty in expressing a diagnosis and treatment plan
- Negative emotional response from provider and patient
- Loss of doctor-patient confidentiality if interpreter is used.

Nevertheless, as for this last point, I should say that it shows a lack of knowledge on the part of some healthcare professionals regarding the profession of the interpreter, and it also indicates the use of *ad hoc* interpreters (not necessarily professional interpreters) in many situations.

Nonetheless, every day there are new studies within the health sciences field related to the topic of providing health care to the migrant community. This has also been the driving force behind the development of new disciplines such as transcultural psychiatry and transcultural medicine and nursing.

Box 1.15.

This development of new disciplines such as transcultural psychiatry and transcultural medicine and nursing is fostered by the respect that is shown in the sciences for ethnic differences. Starting with that perspective, research is conducted to discover how to acquire, develop and secure knowledge and specific skills and techniques so that doctor-patient contact can be efficient in both directions (patient / doctor), even when there is no shared culture in common.

We are, therefore, approaching the territory of transcultural medicine, an area of formal and practical study based in both the humanities and the sciences. Transcultural medicine is focused on the similarities and differences between cultures with regards to healthcare and illness, taking into account possible differences in values in terms of culture, beliefs and behavior in order to provide specific, culturally congruent care.

Lack of communication owing to an insufficient command of a country's official language is perhaps one of the most influential factors, but also one that has been least developed. However, it is something that is receiving more and more mention in guides and publications. The words of Gargantilla (2003: 5) can serve as an example. He clearly states some steps to follow:

- Guarantee migrant access to health care by eliminating all types of barriers and favoring communication.
- Offer information in the native language of the migrant or visitor patient, if necessary through healthcare agents or mediators of the same ethnicity of the patient, or through interpreters.

Given the importance of this topic, I will dedicate the next chapters to explore the topic of linguistic communication with the migrant population.

Practice

This section contains activities to reinforce the information provided in the previous section. The activities can be grouped into two main types: activities for reflection and assimilation of content and activities directed towards research, implementation of skills and strategies in multilingual settings. These activities can be undertaken individually, in pairs or small groups and / or with people from different cultural backgrounds to provide fertile grounds for discussion in class or via email. This will depend largely on the way the book is used (e.g. for self-study, as a textbook, or as support material for any course connected with intercultural communication).

Activity 1.

Look for 2-3 studies on intercultural communication and make a brief summary.

Activity 2.

Look for information on non-verbal communication and mention 2-3 cases that have resulted in conflictive situations or misunderstandings. You can draw from your own experience.

Activity 3.

Find a bibliographic reference and look up the definition of paralanguage. Provide an example (Poyatos 1993, 1976; Candlin and Candlin 2003; Helman, C. 1990).

Activity 4.

Define or look up information on transcultural psychiatry, transcultural medicine, or transcultural nursing. What role does culture play? Is the importance of language mentioned?

Activity 5.

Think about your environment and write about a kind of cultural practice that you feel social workers, doctors, judges, teachers, i.e. potential service providers, may need to know about migrants and visitors that they are not already familiar with or that may seem strange to them.

Activity 6.

Write about some cultural practices or customs that you have observed in hospitals, courts, banks, supermarkets, schools, etc. that you think may be (or are) new or difficult to understand for people who are not familiar with this environment.

Activity 7.

Exchange your answers with other people or discuss the topic with people that you know that have contact with migrant or visitors.

Bibliographic references and further reading

Achotegui, J. (2000). "Los duelos de la migración". In Perdiguero, E. and Comelles, J. M. (Eds.) *Medicina y Cultura.* Barcelona: Editorial Bellaterra, 88-100.

—. (2002). "Immigrants living in extreme situation: immigrant syndrome with chronic and multiple stress (the Ulysses syndrome)". http://www.fhspereclaver.org/migra-salut-mental/Ulises/Ulysses%20text%202%20english-1.pdf [Last accessed April 19th, 2014].

—. (2002). *La Depresión en los Inmigrantes: Una Perspectiva Transcultural*. Barcelona: Ediciones Mayo, S.A.

Alonso, A.; Huerga, H. and Morera, J. (2003). *Guía de Atención al Inmigrante*. SMMFYC. Madrid: Ergon.

Cambridge, J. (1999). "Information loss in bilingual medical interviews through an untrained interpreter". *The Translator*, 5(2) 201-220.

—. (2013). "Working effectively through a professional interpreter." http://publicserviceinterpreting.com/category/public-service-providers/guidance-on-working-effectively-with-interpreters/ [Last accessed April 30th, 2014].

Candlin, C. and Candlin, S. (2003). "Health care communication: A problematic site for applied linguistics research". *Annual Review of Applied Linguistics* 23, 134-154.

Carballo, M. (2006). *El Impacto de la Migración en la Salud: El Caso de la Diabetes*. Centro Internacional para la Migración y la Salud. Encuentro en la Escuela de Verano de Salud Pública.

Clyne, M. (1994). *Inter-cultural Communication at Work: Cultural Values in Discourse*. Cambridge: Cambridge University Press.

Corsellis, A. (2005). "Training Interpreters to work in the Public Services." In Tennent, M. (Ed.) *Training for the New Millennium:*

Pedagogies for Translation and Interpreting. Amsterdam/Philadelphia: John Benjamins, 153-173.
Creeze, I. (2013). *Introduction to Healthcare for Interpreters and Translators*. Amsterdam/Philadelphia: John Benjamins.
Diaz-Cuellar, A., Ringer, H. and Schoeller-Diaz, D. (2013). "The Ulysses syndrome: migrants with chronic and multiple stress symptoms and the role of indigenous linguistically and culturally competent community health workers."
http://www.panelserver.net/laredatenea/documentos/alba.pdf
[Last accessed: April 19th, 2014].
Fernando, S. (Ed.) (1995). *Mental Health in a Multi-ethnic Society*. London and New York: Routledge.
Gargantilla, P. (2003). *Manual de Atención al Inmigrantes*. Madrid: Ergon.
Gumperz, J. (1982). *Discourse Strategies*. Cambridge: Cambridge University Press.
Helman, C. (1990). *Culture, Health and Illness* 2. Oxford: Butterworth - Heinemann.
Kareen J. and Littlewood, R. (1992). *Intercultural Therapy*. Oxford: Blackwell Science.
López Izquierdo, R.; Martín del Barco, O. and Álvarez, P. (2007). *Entrevista al Paciente Inmigrante.* Madrid: AMF, 3(5), 259-266.
Lopez-Velez, R. (2002). *Inmigración y Salud. Aproximación desde Atención Primaria.* Madrid: PBM, SL.
Martincano Gómez J. L. (2004). *Competencia Cultural en la Atención al Inmigrante. Talleres de Práctica Clínica en AP*. Madrid: SCM.
Martincano Gómez, J. L. and García Campayo, J. (2004). *La Salud Mental en el Paciente Inmigrante.* Madrid: IMC.
Martincano Gómez, J. L. (2003). *Manual de Medicina Transcultural*. Madrid: IMC.
Pöchhacker, F. and Kadric, M. (1999). "The hospital cleaner as healthcare interpreter: A case study". *The Translator*, 5(2), 161-178.
Poyatos, F. (1993). *Paralanguage: A Linguistic and Interdisciplinary Approach to Interactive Speech and Sounds.* Amsterdam/Philadelphia: John Benjamins.
—. (1976). *Beyond Words: Theory and Methodology of Nonverbal Communication.* New York: New York State English Council, (NYSEC Monographs, 15).
Sánchez-Reyes, S. and Martín Casado, M. (2005). "Argumentos a favor de la implantación de un servicio de intérpretes en los hospitales". In Valero-Garcés, C. (Ed.) *Traducción como Mediación entre Lenguas y*

Culturas. Translation as Mediation or How to Bridge the Cultural Gap. Alcalá de Henares: Servicio de Publicaciones de la Universidad de Alcalá.

Scollon, R. and Scollon, S. W. (1995). *Intercultural Communication*. Oxford: Blackwell.

Soriano, G. (2002). "La interpretación social en las instituciones hospitalarias de irlanda del norte". In Valero-Garcés, C. and Mancho, G. (Eds.) *Traducción e Interpretación en los Servicios Públicos: Nuevas Necesidades para Nuevas Realidades*, 189-194.

Taibi, M. and Valero-Garcés, C. (2004). "Análisis de la interacción comunicativa en contextos institucionales entre proveedores de servicios, usuarios e intermediarios lingüísticos". *Oralia*, 7, 207-228.

Talero Martín, S. (1997). "La entrevista clínica". In Gil, V. F., Merino, J. and Quirce, F. (Eds.) *Manual de Metodología de Trabajo en Atención Primaria*. Alicante: Universidad de Alicante, 321-34.

Valero-Garcés, C. and Sales, D. (2005). "Translating for new multicultural realities: The complex nature of Translating as a socio-cultural practice". *JOSTRANS*, 7. http://www.jostrans.org/issue07/issue07_toc.php [Last accessed April 30th, 2014].

Valero-Garcés, C. (2004). "Barreras lingüísticas en la comunicación intercultural. Datos y acciones". *Ofrim* 11, 17-36.

—. (2005). "Doctor-patient consultations in dyadic and triadic exchanges". *Interpreting* 7(2), 193-210.

CHAPTER TWO

COMMUNICATING IN MULTILINGUAL SETTINGS

Key Points

- Main concepts related to communication in multilingual settings
- The chain of communication
- Types of encounters in medical consultations
- Misunderstandings when communicating with speakers of other languages
- Conditioning factors that prevent quality in communication
- Key points for the future

Key Readings

Angelelli, C. (2004). *Medical Interpreting and Cross-cultural Communication*. Cambridge: Cambridge University Press.

Pöchhacker, F. & Kadric, M. (1999). "The hospital cleaner as healthcare interpreter: A case study". *The Translator*, 5(2), 161-178.

Davidson, B. (2000). "The interpreter as institutional gatekeeper: the Social-linguistic role of interpreters in Spanish-English medical discourse". *Journal of Sociolinguistics*, 4(3), 379-405.

Valero-Garcés, C. (2005). "Doctor - patient consultations in dyadic and triadic exchanges". *Interpreting*, 7(2), 193-210.

2.1. Introduction. Main concepts related to communication in multilingual settings

This chapter is devoted to an analysis of the elements which play a role in the chain of linguistic communication, the different types of encounters that occur in medical consultations and the problems that arise. As a practical illustration, I will report the outcomes of various studies, with real-life examples of conversations from medical encounters. I share these outcomes to ultimately offer some solutions for the future. Special emphasis is placed on the figure of the intermediary, or third person who acts as a link in the chain of communication. It is this person who makes it possible to overcome the difficulties posed when communicating across different languages and cultures.

I will begin by briefly defining several concepts that are often used when communicating between languages and that have several meanings depending on what context they are used in and by whom. At this stage the book by Bancroft and Rubio-Fitzpatrick´s (2011) *The Community Interpreter* is a useful resource:

> "A" language: The interpreter's primary or native language.
> "B" language: The interpreter's second working language (i.e., his or her second-strongest language)
> "C" language: The interpreter's third working language (i.e., his or her third-strongest language)

"A" language and "B" language vs. L1, L2: The terms "A" Language, "B" Language and "C" Language are traditionally used in translator training institutions, where they indicate the language that the trainee has nominated as their primary or strongest language (A), and the languages they have learnt or in which they need more training (B and C). Generally, interpreters use these terms in the way described above when naming their working languages. On the other hand, the terms "L1", "L2", "L3", and so on are used in the study of language acquisition, sometimes to indicate the *order* in which languages are acquired, and more normally to separate the primary or 'mother' tongue from the others. Although the two nomenclatures often overlap (the trainee's A language is usually their L1), there is a certain logic in separating the criteria of language acquisition from those of translator training.

Ad hoc interpreter is and untrained person who is called upon to interpret, such as a family member interpreting for her parents, a bilingual staff member pulled away from other duties to interpret, a self-declared bilingual in a hospital waiting-room who volunteers to interpret, or an advanced language student; also so called a *chance interpreter* or a *lay interpreter*.

Adjunct interpreter (also known as dual role): A bilingual employee called upon to interpret on occasion or part-time as one of his or her professional duties

Bilingual: A person who is capable of communicating in two languages and who has two different levels of mastery in each language. There are individuals who possess a similar command in both languages and others who show greater skill in one language or specific field. Bilingual is not a synonym of translator or interpreter.

Community interpreter (also known as Public Service Interpreter): a professional interpreter, also frequently refers to bilingual staff members or volunteers who interpret for community services such as health care, education and social services.

Community interpreting (or Public Service Interpreting and Translation): A profession that facilities access to community services (health, police, school…) for linguistically diverse clients who do not speak the language in which the services are offered.

Consecutive interpreting: Rendering a message into another language when the speaker or signer pauses.

Cultural awareness: Recognition of the importance of cultural differences.

Cultural competence: The ability to provide services effectively across cultures.

Cultural sensitivity: A willingness to accept and value cultural differences.

Healthcare interpreting: Interpreting that takes place in any healthcare setting, including, but not limited to: hospitals, community health centers, doctor's offices, health departments, clinics and wellness services; also known as Medical interpreting

Intercultural communication: Relationship, type of contact, interaction or communication among groups of people from different cultures. Interculturality is associated with:

1. Problems resulting from deficient communication (due to a lack of knowledge of the other person's culture) in varied projects and programs: health, education, industry, etc.
2. Problems related to discrimination against persons of diverse racial backgrounds and ethnic groups, and
3. Typically asymmetrical relationships between different cultural and ethnic groups.

Interpreter: A professional who is capable of transferring an oral message from one language to another while keeping the same meaning. This means that the interpreted speech will produce the same effect on the listener as it would on someone listening to the original message in the original language.

Interpreting: The transfer of an oral message from one language to another oral message in a different language so as to create the same effect that was produced in the first language.

Liaison interpretation: A two-way manner of interpreting used to facilitate understanding between two parties that speak different languages. Some authors see liaison interpretation as a type of consecutive interpretation and some experts also call it bilateral interpreting.

Linguistic communication: A complex system of linguistic, cognitive, and sociocultural elements which require great skill on the part of the participants.

Mediation: Any act or utterance of the interpreter that goes beyond interpreting or that takes place outside of the session and that is intended to remove a linguistic barrier to communication.

Sight Translation: The oral or signed translation of a written document into another language. (For example, an interpreter read aloud an informative brochure to the patient.)

Simultaneous interpreting: Rendering a message into another language while the person is still speaking or signing the message.

Source language: The language from which an interpreter interprets at any given moment.

Summarization: Rendering the gist of a message into another language.

Target Language: The language into which an interpreter interprets at any given moment.

Translator: A professional who is capable of transferring a message written in one language into another language while keeping the same meaning. This means that the translated text will have the same effect on the reader as the original message would have on someone reading it in the source language.

Translation: The transfer of a written text in one language to a written text in another language different than that the source language. (SL).

Working languages: The languages into and from which one interprets.

2.2. Communication chain: Possibilities and consequences

Now that the meaning behind these concepts has been clarified, let's return to the topic of communication. Undoubtedly, we all will have observed that communicating with isolated words or making use of a literal translation by focusing only on the meaning found in the dictionary is no guarantee of successful communication. What's more, we forget about strategic components (that allow us to adapt our message to a given situation) and psychomotor skills (produce–receive).

Among the difficulties which have been thoroughly analyzed over the course of previous pages, one topic that has been mentioned on several occasions is that of having no language and culture in common. The following pages will be dedicated to the discussion of intercultural communication from the perspective of the professional who serves as a link between different languages and cultures.

Furthermore, this is something that most speakers have experienced, even when both speakers belong to the same linguistic and cultural community. There are times when misunderstandings will arise or false expectations will be raised; even among friends, because we have not "understood correctly". This risk increases considerably when the participants in the conversation do not share a common language, culture, or either one of the two, or when they are only shared at a very basic or incomplete level. This is a frequent reality for many of the foreign patients in healthcare.

From a linguistic point of view, there are several kinds of encounters that can occur during the medical consultation:

Monolingual encounters:

1. Healthcare staff + patient who barely speaks the official language.
2. Healthcare staff who speak other languages + patient who does not speak official language.

Bilingual encounters:

3. Healthcare staff + patient who does not speak the official language + another adult who accompanies patient.
4. Healthcare staff + patient who does not speak the official language + a child who accompanies patient.

Each one of these participants has a role to play, thus making each medical consultation a singular event. Why is this? It will be explained below.

Box 2.1.

The chain of knowledge transfer in health care begins with the research laboratories in university departments, research institutes and health care companies, where new research knowledge is generated. From there it moves through peer-reviewed publications to the global community. The chain can be broken at any link because of technical, social or fiscal problems, but if the primary link between original researchers and users is broken, nothing new can emerge to support the health services around the world. The global investment made in research is wasted. "The chain of communication in health science: from researcher to health worker through open access" by L. Chan, S. Arunachalam, and B Kirsop, (2009). *Open Medicine*, 3(3), http://www.openmedicine.ca/article/view/298/245 [Last accessed April 30th, 2014].

2.3. Changes in comprehension and expression: outcomes

I will begin by discussing the most frequent causes of misunderstandings with patients who do not speak the content language. Three causes seem to stand out:

- Patient does not speak or understand the official language.
- Patient is not familiar with the culture (and as a result of this, is not familiar with the inner-workings of institutions or the healthcare system.)
- Healthcare staff is not familiar with the patient's culture.

All of the above generates different responses in each one of the participants, as the following chart (Box 2.2) illustrates:

Box 2.2.

Feeling of abuse

Patient $\Leftarrow$ **Staff** $\Rightarrow$

Segregation

The results of some of the research conducted by the Research group FITISPos (Formación e Investigación en Traducción e Interpretación en los Servicios Públicos/*Training and Research in Public Service Translation and Interpreting*) group in Spain (Valero-Garcés 2001, 2004, Lázaro 2010) without a doubt confirm the experience of many healthcare professionals in some regions of Spain at the beginning of the 21st century; an experience that can certainly be observed in other areas as well. It is worth pointing out that in Spain's central region (Madrid and the surrounding region) an elevated percentage of healthcare professionals have cared for patients whose native language is not Spanish; though they claim to have been able to make themselves understood using simplified Spanish and aided by the use of gestures and the assistance of third parties. That said, there is also a relatively high percentage of professionals who feel that neither the patient nor the professional understand the conversations in their totality and as a consequence:

- More time is invested in speaking with the patients
- There is little possibility of obtaining information from the patients
- There is insufficient provision of therapy or the service being sought

With respect to patients, the research conducted by Iliescu (2005) on Romanians in Spain offers interesting data. The belief exists that this group has less difficulty communicating due to certain linguistic and cultural similarities with the Spanish community which facilitate the learning of Spanish and integration into Spanish culture. According to the results of those Romanians surveyed, their level of knowledge in Spanish is good in terms of comprehension (47.1%) and reading (54.7%). However, only 7% believe that this knowledge of Spanish is sufficient to hold one's own in official institutions, while 90% claim to have difficulty. In terms of the availability of information written in the Romanian language, only 4% responded that this information was made available at some point and 96% say that such information was never available. Likewise, when responding to the question if they had ever had the opportunity to receive the help of a mediator or interpreter, 96% said they never had and only 4% responded that they had received this service at some point.

Finally, with respect to the person (family, friend, volunteer) who frequently serves as an intermediary in medical consultations and encounters where there is no common language, the research reveals that these intermediaries also have difficulties communicating. Just an example from a study conducted in 2005 (Valero-Garcés 2005):

> 63.6% said they had problems understanding the speakers.
> 60% indicated difficulties due to a lack of technique or skills necessary to do the job.
> 55% had problems understanding technical language or specific registers and interpreting them.
> 50% admitted to having difficulty deciding on the most appropriate way to address the person.
> 52% felt pressure or impatience from staff.
> 45% mentioned a lack of familiarity with the situation.
> 22.7% felt affected due to anguish or anxiety and due to the anxiety of the patient.

The consequences are not difficult to predict, as referenced by studies: withdrawal from treatment, feelings of uncertainty, distrust, no check-ups, not showing up to medical appointments, etc.

Extracts from real-life conversations taken from recordings of medical consultations illustrate the reality of the situation. This material makes up part of a more extensive corpus of conversations and medical interviews with migrant obtained by the FITISPos group. This data has been collected over the course of many years of research on the quality of the communication with the foreign populations and experience in translators and interpreters' training. An example of different situations follows:

Box 2.3.

*Example 1: (Monolingual conversation 1): **
Doctor (D) + Patient who speaks a little Spanish (P).
Context: Bulgarian patient who is able to speak and understand Spanish with difficulty:
1 D: Se puede tomar todos los días pastilla gorda... hay que ir bajando ¿eh? Entonces, la semana que viene .. esta semana, a partir de mañana...la gorda... las pastillas son así [drawing on a sheet of paper] Esto lo quitas y cortas un trozo ¿entiendes bien? *[Every day you can take big pill... you have to keep reducing it, okay? Then, next week, this week, starting in the morning...the big one...the pills are like this [drawing on a sheet of paper] You take off this and you cut off a piece, do you understand?]*
2 P: [mueve la cabeza de arriba abajo] *[nods head up and down]*

3 D: Y lo guardas... Pasado, el sábado, cortas otro trozo y lo guardas *[And you put it away...the day after, Saturday, you cut off another bit and you put it away]*
4 P: Sí, sí, todo día uno solo, y lo guardo... noche no *[Yes, yes, all day only one and I put it away...not night]*
5 D: Noche no tomar, solo por la mañana ¿vale? Mira esto [enseñando el dibujo]. El domingo, este trozo y este trozo que has guardado te lo tomas ¿eh? Así todos los días... Vamos a bajar poco a poco. *[Night no take, only in the morning, okay? Look at this [showing the drawing]. Sunday, this bit and this bit that you have put away, you take it, okay? Just like that everyday... We're going to lower it little by little.]*

* The translation offered is a literal one, trying to represent "mirror images" of the broken sometimes non-sense Spanish in the original.

The analysis of Example 1 reveals a simplification of the doctor's language and his adaptation of the language to the patient's level of understanding, a lack of command of the language on the part of the patient, and the use of extralinguistic elements such as drawings and body language. The nodding of the head is important, especially if we keep in mind that for Bulgarians, nodding the head up and down indicates a negative response rather than an affirmative one as it does in Spanish.

Box 2.4.

Example 2: (Monolingual conversation 2):

Doctor who speaks (claims to speak) other languages (English or French) on a general level (D) + Patient who speaks a little Spanish (P) + Nurse (N).

Context: Nigerian patient who has problems with pregnancy and a doctor who knows some English.

1 N: ¿Has entendido lo que te dijo la doctora, qué íbamos a hacer? *[Did you understand what the doctor told you, what we are going to do?]*

2 P: Sí, me ha dicho (????) *[Yes, she told me (????)]*

3 D: Sí, que ese bebé se ha perdido, ¿verdad? *[Yes, that that baby was lost, right?]*

4 P: (????)

5 D: No, que no funciona. Eso te dijeron, ¿verdad? Que no exactamente, que va a ser un aborto ya. *[No, that it isn't working. They told you that, right? That it's not exactly, that it's going to be a miscarriage.]*

6 P: También (????) *[Too (????)]*

7 D: ¿También qué? *[Too that?]*

8 P: Me han dicho perrat (????) *[They told me perrat (????)]*

9 D: ¿Perrat?, ¿qué es?, ¡ah! ¿De operar dices o...? *[Perrat?, What's that?, oh! Do you mean operating...?]*

10 P: Mira. Me han dicho seperar. *[Look. They told me seperat.]*

11 D: *Sepera*r. No entiendo. Me estás diciendo, ¿qué idioma es "seperar"?, ¿es español?, ¿*seperar*? *[Seperat. I don't understand. You're telling me. What language is "separat"? Is that Spanish? Seperat?]*

12 P: (*in English) Separated. In English is separated.*

13 D:*In English* ¿cómo es?, ¿*siprich? [(In English) What is it?, siprich?]*

14 P: (*in English)* Separate.

15 D: *Sepreich. Seprich.* No sé lo que quiere decir. *Seprich. [Sepreich. Seprich. I don't know what that means.]*

16 P: Seperar en español, ¿no? *[In Spanish it's "Seperar", right?]*

17 D: (*In English) How do you write in English*? *Separit.* ¿Sabes escribir? *[Do you know how to write?]*

18 P: (*In English) In English, separate, something that divides.*

19 D: (*In English)* ¡oh!, *¡separate*!

20 P: (*In English) But I don't know if that wrote the woman is about.*

21 D: (*In English*) No, no. *Separate is* ...eh, *you have this abortion now. Abortion, abortion.*

22 P: *(In English) Abortion.*

23 D: Es decir, *[What that means is,]* (*in English) the gestation is not, no, no longer going on. It's not going on.*

24 P: ¡Ah!, *the baby is not going on.*

Example 2 shows another situation that can arise during medical consultations, the cases where the doctor and the patient use a third language –in this case English– in order to communicate. Neither of the two parties is able to speak the language fluently and the conversation thus becomes drawn out and difficult.

Box 2.5.

Example 3: (Bilingual Conversation): Doctor (D) + Patient who does not speak Spanish (P) + accompanying person who is an adult (A). Context: A Moroccan woman who does not speak Spanish comes to the doctor's accompanied by her husband who is the one who speaks in Spanish.

01 P: ملي ما كنشربشي الدوا هادا كيعطيني الحريق للطهر (؟؟؟؟) المعدة هاذا كيعملي المعدة واقيلا

02 A: Cuando no tomar este, tiene el dolor de ... de atrás, de aquí. *[When no take this, she has the pain in...back here, right here.]*

03 D: ¿Esto? Esto es para el estómago *[This? This is for her stomach]*

04 P: بلحاق ملي كنشرب هادو (؟؟؟؟)

05 A: Cuando tomar este, tiene el dolor. Siempre quieres este con este, ¿me entiendes? *[When take this, she get the pain. You always want this with this. You understand me?]*

06 D: Ya, a ver, esto es para el *tiroides* para el (¿????) y esto para el *estómago*. *[Okay, let's see, this is for her thyroid for the (¿????) and this for her stomach.]*

07 A and P: Sí *[Yes]*

08 A: Sí, sí *[Yes, yes.]*

09 A: El estómago. *[Her stomach.]*

10 D: ¿Va bien? ¿Bien? *[Is it going okay? okay?]*

11 A: Sí, sí *[Yes, yes.]*

12 D: ¿Sin problemas? Y ¿dónde duele? *[Without any problems? And where does it hurt?]*

13 P: قلو فسنسول دطهري

14 A: Aquí de espalda. *[Here of back.]*

15 D: Pero aquí es distinto, es diferente, distinto al tiroides y al estómago. Esto es otra cosa, diferente, ¿Lo entiende? *[But here is very different, it's different, different from the thyroid and stomach. This is another thing, different. Do you understand?]*

16 A: هاداكشي ما شي هادشي هادا، يمكن الحريق دشي حاجا أخرى

The third example shows another of the situations that tend to occur during medical consultations when the healthcare staff and the patients do not share the same language. We can see the difficulties the companion has in this instance understanding the doctor as well as during his own intervention, where he takes on other roles which go beyond just being the voice of the patient or the doctor.

Below we raise some questions for reflection:

1. Do you feel that they are really communicating?

2. What risks do you see?
3. Have you ever been in a similar situation?
4. What do you think are possible solutions?
5. Wouldn't it be better to have someone on hand who really speaks the two languages well and who is also familiar with the cultures and the workings of the healthcare system in our country? Could it be a professional in intercultural communication – whether we may call that person an interpreter, mediator, or translator?
6. Shouldn't the healthcare facility have such a resource available or be able to provide this service when requested? Who should provide this resource and what should it be?

And, lastly, a common example from multilingual environments in which there are no professionals in interlinguistic communications to be found (interpreters):

Box 2.6.

*Example 4: Bilingual Conversation 2.*_Doctor (D) + Patient who does not speak Spanish (P) + Child who accompanies patient (CH).
Context: A mother who does not speak Spanish attends the medical consult along with her two children: a 2 year old child with diarrhea and vomiting and her 8 year old daughter who speaks some Spanish. After a long and slow conversation with the child as an interpreter the pediatrician prescribes a soft diet of cooked rice with carrots and grilled chicken. The child gives her mother a literal translation of what the provider has said. Both seem surprised but do not say anything and leave the appointment.

What is important to realize here is that while in English the words "grilled chicken" (Box 2.6.) leave little room for misinterpretation, this is not necessarily so in Spanish (in Spanish, *pollo a la plancha*). This is due to the fact that *plancha* can refer to a grill or griddle, but in different contexts means "iron", as in the one used to iron clothing. Look at the image below and ask yourself what might have happened.

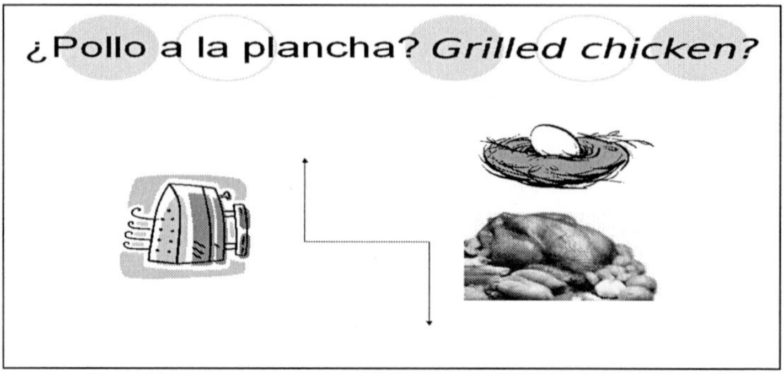

When the mother and her children are leaving, the social worker sees them and asks them how the appointment has gone. The child, without much conviction, replies that it has gone fine and the social worker again asks if anything is wrong. The little girl tells her what the doctor said and that they do not understand how to iron the chicken and then eat it.

If we stop to think for a moment, we realize just how many turns of phrase and fixed expressions a language has that can come up in daily use. This is in addition to the terms that healthcare providers often use that are technical for ordinary speakers and certainly out of reach for a child.

2.4. High quality communication: Triadic healthcare encounters

Beginning with a discussion of certain conditioning factors that prevent quality communication from occurring, there are four that stand out:

1. Lack of awareness from healthcare staff and those responsible for professions of translator, interpreter and mediator in the healthcare facilities.
2. Lack of professionalism (adequate training, application of the code of ethics) from many of those who accompany patients acting as translators, interpreters or mediators.
3. Lack of knowledge or procedures within healthcare institutions that would enable staff to recognize when a specialist in communication is needed.
4. Lack of cooperation and teamwork between different departments or entities when it comes to taking general measures to facilitate communication.

In the following section a brief sketch of each of the points above will follow.

2.4.1. Lack of knowledge about the professions of translator, interpreter and mediator

Anyone who has traveled to a country without knowing its language may have been able to communicate, but at what level? By the same token, if one is not familiar with the culture, there will be expressions or situations that he or she may not be able to understand or that could lead to misunderstandings. Ultimately, language and culture are inseparable. That said, the communications professional (whether that be an interpreter, translator or mediator) is trained for just this.

On the other hand, the terms "interpreter" and "translator" are frequently confused and the term "translator" or "interpreter" is even applied to people who simply know the official language a little bit better, but who lack any type of training to serve as intermediaries. Or, in other words: Would you be able to read a manual in computing or aeronautical engineering and explain it afterwards or translate it directly into English? Some will say that "reading such a specialized text is not the same thing as a medical appointment where the language is more colloquial." Not true! Many terms are used during medical encounters that are considered to be common or every day terms by healthcare staff or even by Spanish patients, but which are in all respects specialized for the foreign patient or the "bilingual" companion or "*ad hoc* interpreter".

Why when we need to manage a legal matter do we go to a lawyer and not to a law student who also is familiar with the law? Why do we bring our car to the garage when it breaks down? Why do we go to the doctor when we have a health problem? Having said that, why do we not turn to specialists in communication when there is problem with communication due to lack of a common language?

Countries which are more advanced in multicultural matters and which are without any doubt multilingual (Australia, United States, Canada, United Kingdom) have developed resources such as interpreting and translation and / or mediation services available in hospitals as well as other resources (See Proceedings of the *Critical Link Conferences*).

2.4.2. Lack of professionalism

Being bilingual does not necessarily imply that one is a professional in interlinguistic communication. Just as we have commented previously, there is an extended belief that simply being able to communicate in another language or languages immediately makes one a qualified translator or interpreter. The table below shows some of the differences that exist between people who know two or more languages and whom we might call "bilingual" and professional translators and interpreters (Cambridge 2002).

Box 2.7.

BILINGUAL	**TRANSLATOR / INTERPRETER**
May have limited fluency in one of the languages.	Fluency is required in both languages.
Has his / her own voice to intervene, express opinions, etc.	Makes communication possible between other people; identifies differences between different languages and cultures and reproduces the messages of others.
There is no code of conduct or personal principles.	Must observe a code of conduct specific to the profession.
There is no need to be prepared to act as a bridge and the message may be transmitted incompletely, parts may be forgotten or omitted if it is considered unimportant, etc.	Must know proper terminology and the procedures needed to be able to faithfully render the message.
No training has been received on how to treat information or about the strategies used to process and reproduce this information.	Usually has certain training or experience so as to be able to process and retain the message faithfully.
May let him / herself be swayed by certain external conditioning factors when transferring the information (compassion, joy, familiarity) and could cease to remain objective, add personal comments, points of view, etc.	Provides accurate information that has been adapted to the new reality and remains detached from any personal considerations.

A detailed, thoughtful reading of the table surely makes us see the reality that exists in certain countries in which there is no established translating or interpreting service in healthcare facilities.

A professional interpreter has received training that goes beyond having knowledge of the two languages and cultures with which he or she works. This knowledge is not an end in itself, but rather a starting point. The training received prepares the interpreter to know how to transfer information from one language to another by correctly "decoding" the messages and by knowing how much information must be provided beyond the words (oral or written) of the speaker. This involves knowing how to properly decode information from the situation and monitoring the comprehension of both parties during each and every exchange, controlling all variables which may affect these exchanges (gender, power, urgent nature of the work...)

Mastery of these skills means that:

1. Communication will not be reduced to a basic level or to the use of gestures.
2. Professionals will know how to relay information or reach the patient.
3. There will be more contact with other communities or professionals who do not share the same language.
4. Professional risk will be reduced, the quality of patient care will improve and even time and money will be saved.

Without a doubt, the first step is for people to become familiarized with these professionals in interlinguistic communication and the differences between them (an interpreter is not the same thing as a translator or mediator) and to not be distrustful of their profession.

Just as with any profession, interpreters must follow an ethical code which, in this case, is based on four main principles:

Confidentiality: Respect the right of others to private life.
Impartiality: Don't take the side of either one of the parties involved.
Precision / Faithful rendition: Assure that the message is faithful to the original and appropriate within the new cultural context.
Integrity: Be honest with oneself about one's abilities or skills before accepting an interpreting / translation job.

The reality is that, at present, in many countries there are no such professionals in hospitals and one speaks of 'interpreters' and 'translators' or 'mediators' without really knowing that these are different professions or that they are fundamental in multilingual societies, even though, as in the case of Spain, the Spanish Law on Patient Healthcare (Law 41/2002) takes into account the right of the patient to understand what is being said to him.

2.4.3. Lack of knowledge or procedures to recognize when a specialist in communication is needed

Have health providers ever stopped to think why this situation occurs and what the consequences could be? The table below illustrates some of the risks involved when a provider seeks the help of a bilingual person (family, friend, acquaintance, volunteer, etc.) who lacks any kind of specific preparation. (Cambridge 2002: 56)

Box 2.8.

Why is this person used?	**Why should they not be used?**
"It's cheaper"	Cheaper than a lawsuit?
"The patient speaks a little Spanish"	Nervousness, the specific situation, the different culture, fear... - they all get in the way of comprehension. Not to mention the moral and legal problems that could be incurred.
"The healthcare provider speaks a little of the other language"	But how will they talk about complicated concepts such as asylum procedures, informed consents, early diagnosis…?
"I get by making hand movements, gestures, drawings"	Right! But did you know there are no international hand gestures? And that symbols and drawings do not have the same meaning either?
"There are always bilingual people available"	But they are not always impartial nor do they uphold confidentiality or follow the code of ethics that, since they are part of a profession, interpreters do.
"The person accompanying the patient is always willing to help out"	Why is that? Might they not have their own motives? Getting medicine for himself or another person, not passing on important information and taking advantage (e.g. wanting the patient to be put on leave from work in order to take his job).

"It is a person the client knows and that is comforting to the patient"	And, for that reason, much of the information may be lost as it may be assumed to be obvious or considered irrelevant.
"They share the same culture"	But there is always the risk that the information required by the healthcare provider may be omitted or that something is explained from a personal point of view rather than from a cultural standpoint.
"Many times it is the children who are the first members of the family to be bilingual"	Should a parent / patient be placed in a child's power? And can a child understand certain concepts?
"The employees (doctors, residents, nurses, cleaning ladies, students…) are close at hand"	What should these people be doing at that moment? Is the expert's time less costly than a professional interpreter's? And what about the risks?

2.4.4. Lack of cooperation and teamwork

Studies conducted in countries possessing more experience with respect to communication in healthcare settings with patients who do not speak the official language show that there are a series of processes which occur consecutively. Each link making up the chain of communication must undergo these consecutive processes. These links are:

a) The healthcare staff.
b) The patients who do not have a good command of the language in which those services are offered.
c) The intermediaries who make the communication possible.

Each one of these links must undergo a process of change. In the case of public services (within which we include healthcare services), one typically moves through these stages differently and at varying speeds. They are (Corsellis 2002: 182-186):

1. A lack of recognition of the problem.
2. Denial of the problem and attempts to find solutions which often are not very rational. This leads to the typical comments heard so many times in healthcare settings: "We do not usually have problems because they come

with their children or friends who help them", "We are able to understand one another with gestures, drawings...", "There are people in the clinic who can lend a hand if necessary."
3. Recognition (accepting the problem).
4. Analysis and implementation of solutions.

This final stage requires a strategy and it is difficult to specify the amount of time this can take. Not only is it necessary to have professionals that can perform the tasks of interpreting and interpreter training, but it is also necessary that healthcare employees receive training to be able to work with people of other cultures or with interpreters. (See Corsellis 2003: 71-90).

There are public services that have managed to implement important resources with positive results both in terms of training as well as in terms of monitoring outcomes or providing multilingual services. This is the case in countries such as Australia, USA, Canada, or Sweden (e.g. healthcare services, court interpretations) though less progress has been made in other areas (education, social services). There can even be great differences between different countries or even between different areas within the same country.

5. Progress made on a local level through personal and private initiatives, after overcoming great difficulties. The most common way the action stage is initiated is after recognizing that there is a problem that needs a solution, through enthusiastic people and committed volunteers. This is what happens in Spain with non-profits.
6. Institutionalization on a national level. Social change comes about differently in different cultures. It may occur at the same time as the passing of laws in the host country or as a consequence thereof or it may come about on the tail of legislative changes that can take place because of the current situation.
7. Consistency on a local level within a national framework after achieving a series of general measures: codes of conduct, professional interpreter services, or interpreters´ associations.

2.5. Key points for a better future

The development of a new society is already in progress and it cannot be denied that we are finally beginning to take action after having progressively become aware of the situation. The guides to caring for the migrant patient written by healthcare professionals and which include recommendations to improve the situation are ever greater in number. In the case of Spanish, some examples are the works by López Velez 2002,

Gargantilla 2003, Martíncano 2003 2004 a,b, or Carballo 2006. Some of the measures indicated are the following:

Box 2.9.

- Eliminating barriers to the exchange of information.
- Search for cooperation and exchange of resources.
- Support for the production of high-quality materials in minority languages and the dissemination of these materials, as well as other resources (network of translators and interpreters, telephone service, etc.).
- Training courses and seminars for healthcare workers, as well as for mediators, translators and interpreters.
- Development of international projects and stepping up research, not only between different communities but also between countries. Migration is a global phenomenon and there are countries which have more experience than Spain.
- Availability of professionals in intercultural communication: trained translators, interpreters, and intercultural mediators. This is not just someone who is bilingual, who may have difficulties in one of the languages, may not know specific vocabulary, does not adhere to ethical principles, does not master the basic techniques involved in the transfer of information from one language to another and who may fill more roles than just that of interpreter: companion, spouse, nurse, doctor, lawyer…
- Teamwork

Cooperation and teamwork are some of the recommendations from experts. All parties -service providers as well as users- must be involved in the process. In this regard, we must acknowledge the fact that the situation is also changing for public service employees, who must work with people who speak other languages and come from different cultures. Therefore, the need to adapt to such change will clearly have to be combined with a wide range of variables.

Ann Corsellis (2003: 71) lists the characteristics or skills that professionals working in such environments must have or which need to be developed:

1. Communication skills.
2. The ability to put professional skills into practice.
3. Connections with other disciplines within the team and public.
4. Work ethics.

This clearly and specifically implies that the linguistic intermediaries or this third element that helps communicate must:

1. Be familiar not only with the language but also with the culture in order to correctly "decode" messages and know which information must be transferred with more than just words (either spoken or written).
2. Properly decode the message according to the situation.
3. Make sure that the parties understand one another, coordinating all the variables that may affect communication (sex, power, urgency of the work, etc.).

As Corsellis points out, mastery of these skills will:

1. Prevent communication from being reduced to gestures or to a basic level.
2. Allow professionals to understand how to properly transmit information to the service user.
3. Increase contact with other communities or professionals who do not share the same language.
4. Reduce occupational risks, improve the quality of user care, and even save time and money.

Acknowledging these facts has lead to the development of proposals in specialized settings.

Currently some of these recommendations have been put into practice in some countries and hopefully more actions will be taken.

2.6. Summary

In order to summarize what has been said up until now and to simplify the situation which still occurs in many healthcare centers and hospitals in which different languages and cultures coexist, we present the following table (Box 2.10):

Box 2.10.

Constant flow of migrant population to healthcare centers
↓
New challenges and problems
↓
Greater effort and new difficulties for professionals in their work
↓
Search for solutions.

Practice

This section contains activities to reinforce the information provided in the previous section. The activities can be grouped into two main types: activities for reflection and assimilation of content and activities directed towards research, implementation of skills and strategies in multilingual settings. These activities can be undertaken individually, in pairs or small groups and / or with people from different cultural backgrounds to provide fertile grounds for discussion in class or via email. This will depend largely on the way the book is used (e.g. for self-study, as a textbook, or as support material for any course connected with intercultural communication).

Activity 1.

Debate:
1. Considering some of the factors mentioned that may condition quality in communication, what is the situation in you country / area?
2. What mechanisms for collaboration are offered by institutions?
3. What resources are there?
4. Is there a group of translators and interpreters in your workplace?
5. Is there training available to healthcare professionals regarding intercultural communication and the importance of language?
6. Do medical professionals receive training on how to work with interpreters?

Activity 2.

Reflect upon the dialogue excerpts from the medical encounters which were mentioned above and think about your own experience or about that of your colleagues and try to answer the following questions or to imagine the following situation:

1. Do the participants manage to communicate easily?
2. Would you say that the communication is first-rate?
3. What types of problems do you think each of the participants might have: doctor-patient-intermediary?
4. How might they be resolved?
5. What consequences do you think might result when there is not complete understanding?
6. What would be the ideal medical encounter?

Activity 3.

Base on the outcomes of some of the research presented here or on your own experience, please reflect:

1. Do you think that the patients are able understand and that they go home feeling convinced of what they have been told?
2. What consequences do you foresee? Withdrawal from treatment, feeling unsure, distrust.....?
3. Do you have any personal experience in this?
4. If possible, exchange comments with other colleagues.

Bibliographic references and further reading

Bancroft, M and Rubio-Fitzpatrick, L. (2011). *The Community Interpreter.* Columbia, US: Cross-Cultural Communications.

Cambridge, J. (1999). "Information loss in bilingual medical interviews through an untrained interpreter". *The Translator,* 5(2), 201-219.

__. (2002). "Interlocutor roles and the pressures as interpreters". In Valero-Garcés, C. and Mancho, G. (Eds.) *Traducción e Interpretación en los Servicios Públicos: Nuevas Necesidades para Nuevas Realidades / New Needs for New Realities.* Alcalá de Henares: Servicio de Publicaciones de la Universidad, 121-126.

—. (2003). "Unas ideas sobre la interpretación en los centros de salud." In Valero-Garcés, C. (Ed.) *Traducción e Interpretación en los Servicios Públicos. Contextualización, Actualidad y Futuro.* Granada: Comares, 57-59.

Cordella, M. (2004). *The Dynamic Consultation: A Discourse Analytical Study of Doctor–Patient Communication* (Vol. 128). Amsterdam / Philadelphia: John Benjamins.

Corsellis, A. (2003). "Formación de los proveedores de servicios públicos para trabajar con intérpretes y traductores. Habilidades y competencias interculturales". *Traducción e Interpretación en los Servicios Públicos. Contextualización, Actualidad y Futuro.* Granada: Comares, 71-90.

—. (2006). "Making sense of reality." *Linguistica Antverpiensia, Special issue: Taking stock: research and methodology in community interpreting,* 341-352.

—. (2005). "Training interpreters to work in the Public Services". In Tennent, M. (Ed.) *Training for the New Millennium: Pedagogies for Translation and Interpreting.* Amsterdam / Philadelphia: John Benjamins, 153-173.

Davidson, B. (2000). "The interpreter as institutional gatekeeper: the Social-linguistic role of interpreters in Spanish-English medical discourse". *Journal of Sociolinguistics,* 4(3), 379-405.

Gargantilla Madera, P. (2003). *Manual de Atención a Inmigrantes.* Madrid: Ergon.

Illiescu, C. (2006). "Sentido y sensibilidad en el papel del intérprete social en ámbito médico-sanitario en la Provincia de Alicante". *Actas del XXIV Congreso de AESLA celebrado en la UNED.* Madrid, 29-30 marzo de 2006.

Kaufert, J. and Putsch, R. (1997). "Communication through interpreters in healthcare: Ethical dilemmas arising from differences in class, culture, language and power". *The Journal of Clinical Ethics*, 8(1), 71-87.

Lázaro Gutiérrez, R. (2010). *Análisis del discurso institucional entre hablante nativo (HN) y hablante no nativo (HNN) en los servicios públicos*. [Unpublished doctoral dissertation]. Universidad de Alcalá, Madrid, Spain.

López-Vélez, R. and Huerga, H. (2002). *Inmigración y Salud. Aproximación Desde Atención Primaria*. Madrid: PBM.

Marticano Gómez, J. L., Rodríguez, V. M. G., Correales, R. G. and Campayo, J. G. (2004). *Los Problemas de Salud Mental en el Paciente Inmigrante*. Madrid: IMC.

Martincano Gómez, J.L. (2003). *Manual de Medicina Transcultural.* Madrid: IMC.

Mesa, A. M. (2000). "The cultural interpreter: An appreciated professional. Results of a study on interpreting services: client, health care worker and interpreter points of view". In Roberts, R., Carr, S.E., Abraham D. and Dufour, A. (Eds.) *The Critical Link 2: Interpreters in the Community*. Amsterdam / Philadelphia: John Benjamins, 67-79.

Ong, L., De Haes, J., Hoos, A. and Lammes, F. (1995). "Doctor-patient communication: a review of the literature". *Social Science and Medicine*, 40(7), 903-918.

Ozolins, U. (1998). *Interpreting and Translating in Australia: Current Issues and International Comparisons,* Melbourne: Language Australia.

Pöchhacker, F. and Kadric, M. (1999). "The hospital cleaner as healthcare interpreter: A case study". *The Translator*, 5(2), 161-178.

Valero-Garcés, C. (2005). "Doctor-patient consultations in dyadic and triadic exchanges". *Interpreting,* 7(2), 193-210.

Valero-Garcés, C., and Martin, A. (Eds.). (2008). *Crossing Borders in Community Interpreting: Definitions and Dilemmas* (Vol. 76). John Benjamins Publishing.

CHAPTER THREE

CHANGES IN THE HEALTHCARE SETTING: PERCEPTIONS FROM THE FIELD ABOUT THE USE OF THE LANGUAGE

Key Points

- English as a lingua franca in healthcare settings.
- Resources available at healthcare facilities.
- Perceptions from medical staff about the use of English in healthcare facilities.
- Perceptions from English-speakers about the use of English in healthcare facilities.
- Degree of satisfaction with resources available to communicate with foreign population.

Key Readings

David, R.A., Rhee, M. (1998). "The impact of language as a barrier to effective health care in an underserved urban Hispanic community". *The Mount Sinai Journal of Medicine,* 1998; 65(5-6, 393-397.

Freeman, G. K., Rai, H., Walker, J. J., Howie, J. G. R., Heaney, D. J., Maxwell, M. (2002). "Non-English speakers consulting with the GP in their own language: A cross-sectional survey". *British Journal of General Practice*. 2002; 52, 36-38.

Lawrenson R, Leydon G, Freeman G, et al. (1998). "Are we providing for ethnic diversity in accident & emergency (A & E) departments?". *Ethnicity & Health.* 1998; 3, 117-123.

Narayanan, A. (2012). "Interpreters may help shorten hospital stays". *Chicago Tribune*. 18th of June, 2012. http://articles.chicagotribune.com/2012-05-25/lifestyle/sns-rt-us-hospital-interpretersbre84o0z4-20120525_1_interpreters-patients-general-internal-medicine [Last accessed April 30th, 2014].

3.1 Introduction

This chapter will center on providing a description of the current state and evolution of healthcare services in a specific country. This is done in order to show what occurs in other countries as they evolve into multicultural societies in which intercultural communication is a necessity.

3.2 The current situation in Spain

Intercultural communication is a fundamental part of modern societies that affects people from all over the world. Cultural intermixing as a result of migration is an inevitable reality for many countries which needs to be addressed and cannot be ignored.

A closer look at the healthcare services in Spain reveals important changes in the structure of a doctor's visit and in the attitude of medical professionals. One of the main causes is the arrival of migrants that bring different languages and cultures and that do not have a good command of the contact language – Spanish in this case.

They are new patients with new needs and they require new solutions. Multidisciplinary efforts and teamwork could provide some solutions, given the disparity of opinions and the lack of knowledge people have of one another. This is true not only among professionals and migrants and visitors, but also within the professions themselves that, in one form or other, assist migrant populations, that is, doctors, nurses, psychologists, social workers, anthropologists, sociologists, educators, foreign language teachers, linguists, translators and interpreters, professionals in administration, teachers and researchers. Some of the examples presented so far show that the quality of communication needs to be improved.

Cultural diversity in Spain is on the rise and is an issue that has changed many aspects of how the country works in regards to public services. This is a comparative study which focuses on how the English-speaking population of Madrid is being affected by language and cultural barriers in healthcare settings following the study by Ashley Krewatch (2012). This chapter and the following one are dedicated to the analysis and comparison of the perspectives of both medical staff and English-speaking residents in the city of Madrid. It is also an example of the need to join theory and research, and as a way to go a step further in the building of a multicultural society.

Healthcare providers in touch with the migrant populations arriving on a daily basis, must realize that they are working in a multicultural environment, and that they need to use adequate resources to facilitate communication, or if not available, they must begin to develop them.

Box 3.1.

> There are increasingly more jobs in the area of public services, where employees work with people of other languages and cultures and also help people with very different needs where the difficulty of the ignorance of the language and the functioning of institutions is added. The need to adapt to the changes and to have or develop resources to help in the communication process is therefore evident.

Ann Corsellis (2003: 71), while enumerating the characteristics that professionals in these settings must possess or develop, speaks about the competence and the professional skills required and about the connections with other disciplines privately and publicly; along with some communication skills and a strong work ethic. The tools required to implement this type of program exist, given that there are countries that have greater experience and that have developed these programs; the fact that service providers can gather information on what has been done in these countries is a major step, at least in the case of the southern and eastern EU countries. They are taking their first steps in shaping a new multicultural society and the decisions that are made today will certainly affect their future.

These countries are still at a stage of raising awareness of this new reality and in the analytical phase of the new requirements generated by this reality. However, the interest in this stage is not widespread, neither in society nor in the different official institutions or their service providers. The fact that this even happens in countries with as much experience as the U.S.A., where there are increasing trans-state scope projects and the volume of translated materials in the healthcare system and within the administration grows by the day. However, there are other areas where less progress has been made, such as education and the quality of the materials that are offered. Therefore, when facing budget cuts, these services are often the first to be reviewed; even though research shows that having good communication networks would lower cost and reduce wasted efforts.

Today, however, the information is scattered; as indicated by the title of this article, it is difficult to gather information in this field. One of the main causes is precisely linguistic: most of the material is written in English, which constitutes an obstacle for many of the employees in public services and the service providers in Spain. On the other hand, a portion of the migrant population that arrives cannot communicate in English either.

3.3 English-speakers' personal comments on survey

Krewatch (2012) in her study "Two sides of the same coin: the perspective of English speaking patients and doctors in Madrid" includes first-hand accounts from English-speaking residents that currently live in Madrid or have done so within the past five years. Therefore, the information provided is regarded as highly valuable because their thoughts and stories help to get a real sense of the current level of satisfaction that English-speaking residents have regarding the health care system in Madrid.

Box 3.2.

Q&A 1: *Which resources are currently being used during medical encounters in order to facilitate communication between healthcare professionals and patients that do not speak Spanish?*

We were also interested in finding out which resources are currently being used during medical encounters in order to facilitate communication between healthcare professionals and patients that do not speak Spanish. Those surveyed had the option of choosing from different resources: educational pamphlets, professional interpreters, friends or family members, gestures, telephone interpreters, or can communicate fluently in several languages.

Data shows the following: Out of 45 people surveyed, 8 (18%) indicated that they have educational pamphlets available in other languages; 4 (9%) use professional interpreters; 34 (76%) communicate through the patient's friends or family members that speak Spanish; 18 (40%) feel that they get by with gestures; 2 (4%) use telephone interpreters; 16 (36%) are able to communicate in several languages; and 16 (36%) chose 'other' and wrote an explanation on the line provided.

Apart from illustrating the data in terms of the total number of people surveyed, we also see a breakdown of the resources used at each healthcare facility (according to each type of facility,) whether private or public. The data shows the number of people who use the resource in question over the total number of participants in each facility. The following are the results from the public facilities: of the 6 people surveyed from the non-specified CMS (Madrid Health Center), 1 communicates with pamphlets, 1 using professional interpreters, 6 with *ad hoc* interpreters, 3 with gestures and 1 chose 'other'. Of the 2 people surveyed from CMS Fuencarral, 1 communicates using pamphlets, 1 with professional interpreters, 2 through *ad hoc* interpreters, 1 with gestures and 1 chose 'other'. The individual surveyed from CMS Retiro communicates through *ad* hoc interpreters and gestures. Of the 8 people surveyed from CMS Usera, 1 communicates using pamphlets, 7 using *ad hoc* interpreters, 4 with gestures and 2 with telephone interpreters. Of the 3 surveyed from CMS Joven, 2 communicate with pamphlets, 2 with *ad hoc* interpreters, 1 with gestures, 1 in other languages and 3 chose 'other'. Of the 4 people surveyed from CMS Villa de Vallecas, 1 communicates with pamphlets, 3 with *ad hoc* interpreters, 2 with gestures, 1 in other languages, and 1 chose 'other'. The individual surveyed from CMS International communicates with *ad hoc* interpreters and gestures. Of the 5 people surveyed from CMS San Blas, 2 communicate with pamphlets, 3 with *ad hoc* interpreters, 2 with gestures, and 2 in other languages.

The following are the results from the private facilities: Of the 3 people surveyed from CM (Medical Clinic) Conde de Orgaz, 1 communicates using *ad hoc* interpreters, 1 with gestures, 3 in other languages and 2 chose 'other'. Of the 7 people surveyed from CM Gran Vía, 1 communicates using professional interpreters, 6 with *ad hoc* interpreters, 2 with gestures, 5 in other languages and 4 chose 'other'. Of the 4 people surveyed from PS (Health Polyclinic) 4 Clinicians, 2 communicate with *ad hoc* interpreters, 3 in other languages and 3 chose 'other'.

Box 3.3.

As Krewatch points out, certain differences can be found between the public facilities and private facilities. The resource which is most frequently used in public facilities is that of *ad hoc* interpreters (friends, family members) (83%) and in private facilities it is one's knowledge of other languages (73%). Among the public facilities, 27% of those facilities had pamphlets available in other languages, but none of the private facilities had this available. The most under-utilized resource in both health care systems was telephone interpreters, although 7% did indicate using this resource.

The majority (10) of the 16 people who chose "other" used the line provided to explain more about their level in other languages apart from English. This could be because the option before "other" is "I can communicate fluently in several languages". Thus, some did not indicate being able to communicate fluently; instead they listed the other languages in which they do have some proficiency. Those who indicated speaking other languages fluently noted which ones. However, 5 of those surveyed mentioned alternative resources that they used that were not among the options provided. These are: the patients come with information written down in English, bilingual dictionary (English) online, *Universal Doctor* online program, patient accompanied by mediator and documents prepared in English. The last person surveyed was not part of the two aforementioned groups (those who described their language level and those that added another resource) and wrote: "none, in Spain we speak Spanish". This person did not choose any of the other options.

The primary resource used during medical encounters, according to this study, is English; both spoken and written.

The following questions are intended to qualify the level of English of each person:

Box 3.4.

Q&A 2: *How would you rate your level in English from 1 to 5? (1-beginner, 5-advanced) 1, 2, 3, 4, 5, I do not speak English.*
Q&A 3: *How often do you use English to facilitate communication with foreign patients? Often, sometimes, seldom, never*
Q&A 4: *Are there materials available to you in English (pamphlets, informed consents, etc.) Yes, Which ones? No.*

The information found in Graph 3.1 shows the level of English of each person surveyed from 0 to 5, as determined by self-evaluation. In each category from 0 to 5, there is a breakdown showing how often English is used in the encounters.

Of the 45 people surveyed, 3 (7%) marked the "I do not speak English" option. Of these 3, all of them (100%) indicated that they never use English as a resource. 7 (15.5%) of those surveyed checked 1. Of these, 5 (71.5%) used English sometimes and 2 (28.5%) never did. 14 (31%) of those surveyed checked 2. Of these, 1 (7%) used it often, 2 (14%) sometimes and 11 (79%) seldom. 13 (29%) of those surveyed marked 3. Of these, 2 (15%) used it often, 4 (31%) sometimes and 7 (54%) seldom. 7 (15.5%) of those surveyed checked 4. Of these, 1 (14%) used it often, 3 (43%) sometimes, 2 (29%) seldom and 1 (14%) never. Lastly, 1 (2%) of those surveyed marked 5 and used English often during medical encounters.

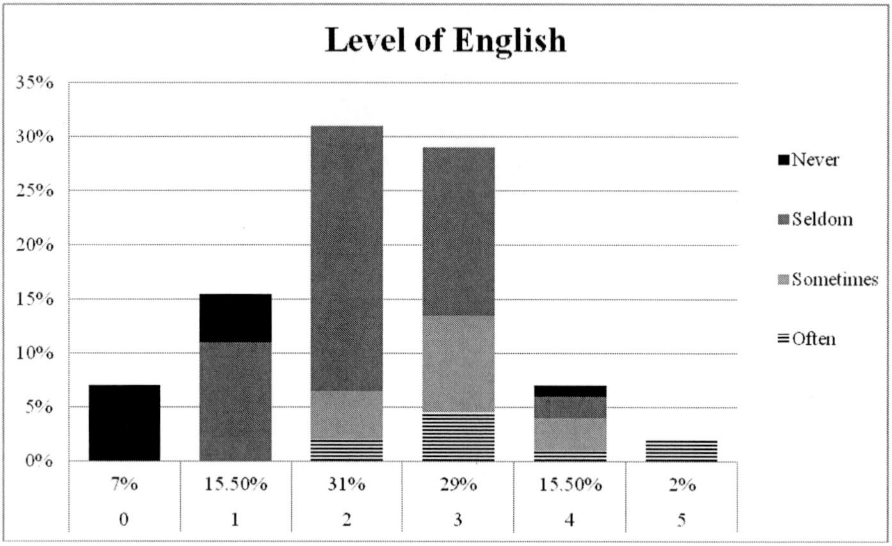

Graph 3.1: Level of English of surveyed and when communicating with foreign patients

The results obtained from question 7 are as follows: 5 (11%) use English often; 9 (20%) sometimes; 25 (55.5%) seldom; and 6 (13.5%) never. This means that if the "seldom" and "never" categories are combined, 31 of those surveyed (69%) do not usually use English as a resource during medical encounters with non-Spanish speaking patients.

Graph 3.2 illustrated the results from question 8. Of 45 people surveyed, 8 (18%) indicated having written materials in English available to them, while those remaining (37 of those surveyed, 82%) indicated that they did not have any written material available in English. On the line provided next to the question "Which ones?", for question 8, were the following answers: HIV; HIV, birth control methods; pamphlets on birth control methods; about other organisms; pamphlets; birth control and HIV/STI, but they are not from Madrid Health; pamphlets about sexual and reproductive health: STI, HIV, birth control; pamphlets. These 8 people work in different branches of the Madrid health care centers, so it is logical that they provide similar answers regarding what materials are available.

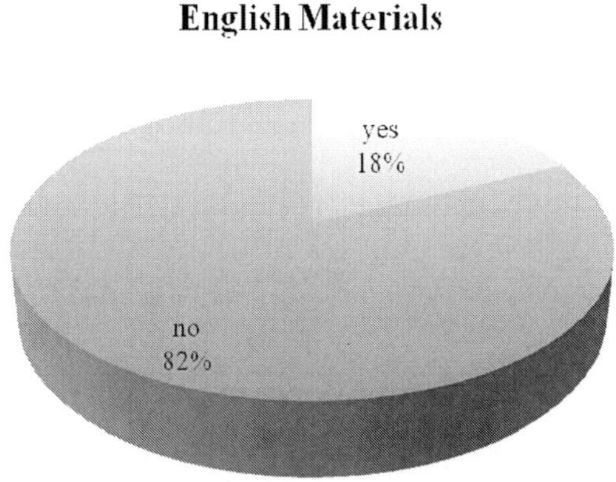

Graph 3.2: Percentage of materials available in English

An interesting detail is that 6 of the 37 people surveyed, who indicated not having materials available in English, checked the option "I have educational pamphlets in other languages available" on question 5. From this information we can conclude that the pamphlets they have are written in languages other than English. The opposite also occurred: 6 of the 8 that indicated having materials available in English did not mark "I have educational pamphlets available in other languages" for that question. This could mean that the materials they do have are not pamphlets or that they are pamphlets but that they do not use them often enough to mark them on question 5. It is also possible that they made a mistake answering the question.

Box 3.5.

Q&A 5: *In general, how would you rate the level of communication between you and the non-Spanish speaking patients from 1 to 5 (1 – no or very little communication, 5 – fluent communication) 1, 2, 3, 4, 5*

Question 5 is the same as the last question on the survey, which is directed at the English speakers. The goal of the question was to obtain a general rating from those surveyed once they had been required take many different elements into consideration while completing previous questions. Table 3.1 shows the rating of the level of communication according to each health care professional surveyed. The ratings are grouped according to the different job titles in the facilities and the last row shows the results for all of those surveyed. In order to provide a clearer idea of what each possible rating means the following words describing the communication have been added in parenthesis: 1 (none / very low), 2 (low), 3 (good), 4 (very good) and 5 (fluid).

Level of communication	1 (none / low)	2 (low)	3 (good)	4 (very good)	5 (fluid)
Doctors	1/9	2/9	4/9	2/9	0/9
Family practitioners	0/8	0/8	2/8	5/8	1/8
Gynecologists	0/3	1/3	1/3	0/3	1/3
Dermatologists	0/1	1/1	0/1	0/1	0/1
Specialists	0/2	0/2	0/2	2/2	0/2
Oftalmologists	0/1	0/1	1/1	0/1	0/1
Endocrinologists	0/1	0/1	1/1	0/1	0/1
Pediatricians	0/6	2/6	1/6	2/6	1/6
Nurses	3/8	1/8	4/8	0/8	0/8
Midwives	0/4	0/4	3/4	1/4	0/4
Social workers	0/1	0/1	1/1	0/1	0/1
Blank answers	1/1	0/1	0/1	0/1	0/1
Total Surveyed	**5/45 (11%)**	**7/45 (15%)**	**18/45 (40%)**	**12/45 (27%)**	**3/45 (7%)**

Table 3.1: Level of communication as rated by health care staff and classified by job title

Of the 9 doctors, 1 marked rating 1, 2 marked 2, 4 marked 3 and 2 marked 4. Of the 8 family practitioners, 2 marked 3, 5 marked 4 and 1 marked 5. The dermatologist marked 2. The 2 medical specialists marked 4. The oftamologist marked 3. The endocrinologist marked 3. Of the 6 pediatricians, 2 marked 2, 1 marked 3, 2 marked 4 and 1 marked 5. Of the 8 nurses, 3 marked 1, 1 marked 3 and 4 marked 3. Of the 4 midwives, 3 marked 3 and 1 marked 4. The social worker marked 3 and the person who left their job title blank marked 1.

In total, 5 of those surveyed (11%) marked 1, 7 (15%) marked 2, 18 (40%) marked 3, 12 (27%) marked 4 and 3 (7%) marked 5. The most common rating was 3, indicating that there is a good level of communication between those surveyed and their non-Spanish speaking patients.

Box 3.6.

Q&A 6: *Are you satisfied with the resources you use to communicate with foreign patients or would you add / eliminate any of the resources you have used up until now? Yes, I am satisfied; No, I would change the following aspects:*____________________

Question 6 is the last question on this survey. This question was aimed at getting the person to consider all the resources that he/she uses, to reflect on them and to decide if they are satisfied or not with these means of communication. If the person was not satisfied, they were asked to explain on the line provided which resources should be changed or added in order to raise their level of satisfaction.

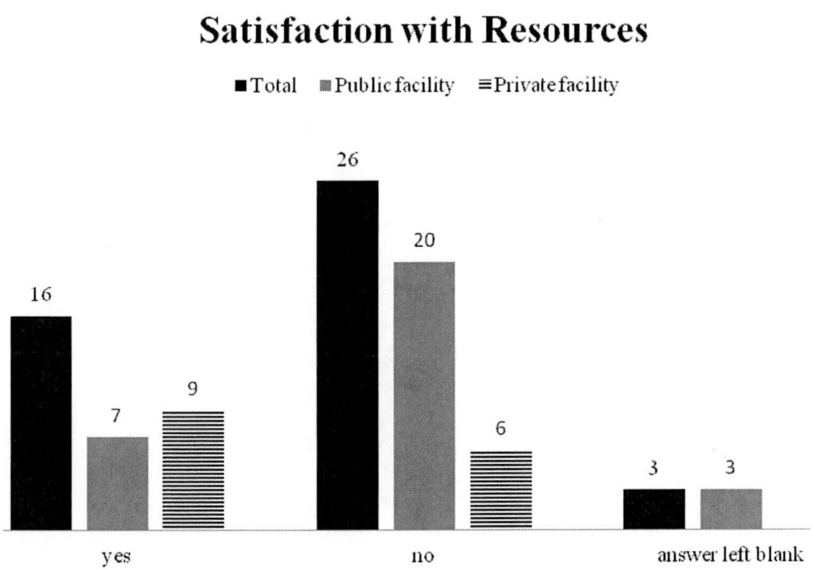

Graph 3.3: Percentage of NSSP satisfied with the resources

Graph 3.3 shows the satisfaction of those surveyed. The three categories on the graph are "yes" and "no" and, since some did not answer the question, "answer left blank". The bars in each category show the data obtained from everyone that took the survey and also grouped by public and private facilities.

The following results were obtained from question 1: 16 (35.5%) of those surveyed indicated that they were satisfied with the resources they used. Of these, 7 (44%) work in a public facility and 9 (56%) in a private one. 26 (58%) indicated they were not satisfied. Of these, 20 (77%) work in a public facility and 6 (23%) in a private one. 3 (6.5%) left the answer blank, all of whom work in a public facility. These results suggest that the majority of those surveyed have a low level of satisfaction with respect to the resources they use. This may be because they don't have access to resources that they feel might be useful. All but 3 of the 26 people surveyed that indicated not being satisfied explained why on the line provided. These comments will be analyzed in Chapter 6 of this study.

3.4. Conclusions

The results of this study lend a deeper perspective on the current situation in terms of the intercultural communication between English-speaking residents and professionals in the healthcare sector in Madrid. The analysis of the data prompted reflection on the methods and tools that are now being used to break the linguistic barriers between these two groups. What follows is a summary of the conclusions drawn from this research along with some suggestions for future improvement. These suggestions are aimed at promoting integration between the foreign and native populations.

Several similarities were found between this study and the studies mentioned in Chapter 1, indicating that there has not been enough positive change to improve the situation for migrants when it comes to healthcare:

- There is still no official medical interpreting service.
- The level of English of Spaniards is generally low.
- In the health care facilities studied, there is a lack of written information about health care in different languages.
- Resources which pose a risk for both health care professionals and patients are overused.
- These resources include machine translation, the use of *ad hoc* interpreters, and communication through gestures.
- These resources are known to pose risks because there is an increased chance of error during the transmission of information from one language to another when they are utilized.

In short, the results of the survey directed at the English-speaking residents shown that the majority of those who had gone to a health care facility did not receive any significant information in English. Through an analysis of the comments of those surveyed, it is clear that the English-speakers have some interest in communicating through written materials.

It has been demonstrated that there are cultural differences between English-speaking people and the Spanish; and in spite of the fact that these differences might not be as striking as the differences between the Spanish and those of certain other cultures; they can still effect the communication between the two groups, especially in a healthcare setting. Given the fact that intercultural communication is not only about linguistics, but also about cultural understanding, it requires the help of someone who possesses knowledge of both of these elements.

This is another reason that the aforementioned overused resources do not usually work so well. Machine translators only provide linguistic assistance and although they do offer limited help, they are not always reliable. It may be true that *ad hoc* interpreters are aware of certain aspects of their own culture and that they are even able to recognize differences between the two cultures involved, but since they are not professionals, they could omit this important information if they are not aware that it is significant for the comprehension between the healthcare professional and patient.

The use of educational pamphlets presents the advantage of allowing the patient to read the information as many times as he / she wants, as the information is always made available. However, apart from offering pamphlets in English, it would also be advisable to offer any type of texts, for example, consent forms in English; given that it is extremely important that everything set forth in such a document be understood. Any misunderstanding or error resulting from a patient's inability to comprehend a document that he/she has signed could lead to serious consequences.

Practice

This section contains activities to reinforce the information provided in the previous section. The activities can be grouped into two main types: activities for reflection and assimilation of content and activities directed towards research, implementation of skills and strategies in multilingual settings. These activities can be undertaken individually, in pairs or small groups and / or with people from different cultural backgrounds to provide fertile grounds for discussion in class or via email. This will depend largely on the way the book is used (e.g. for self-study, as a textbook, or as support material for any course connected with intercultural communication).

Activity 1.

After Reading the chapter, answer the following questions:

1. Which aspect does Corsellis consider relevant to facilitate communication with the foreign population? Do you think these conditions exist in Spain?

2. According to the Spanish *Secretaría General de Inmigración y Emigración*, as of December 31, 2011 there was a total of 5,251,094 foreign residents in Spain. Can you check this data for 2014? Has it changed? Is it lower or higher? If you are from a different country, check the changes in population in the last 3 years or so?

3. According with you own experience, comment upon the results for Q&A 1. Have you visited the same health care facilities in Madrid?

4. If you are a foreign-language speaker, has the healthcare specialist spoken to you in English or in another language? Did it help?

5. If you are a healthcare specialist or work in a hospital, will you talk to your patients in English? Yes? No? At certain times?

Activity 2.

Looking around: have you ever been offered or seen any written material in English or in any other foreign language in a healthcare facility? Look for some examples and provide a short description of what you have found.

Activity 3.

Write a comment for question 6 from your own perspective (medical staff, Spanish patient, or non-Spanish speaking patient). Do you agree with the data provided? What is your own experience?

Activity 4.

List the main aspects that, according to this text, still need to be considered in shaping a Spanish multicultural society. Add any suggestion you may have. If possible, exchange comments with your classmates.

Bibliographic references and further reading

Aerny Perreten N., Ramasco Gutiérrez M., Cruz Maceín J., Rodríguez Rieiro C., Garabato González S. and Rodríguez Laso, A. (2010). "La salud y sus determinantes en la población inmigrante de la Comunidad de Madrid." *Gaceta Sanitaria*, 24(2), 136-144.

Carrasco Garrido, P., Jiménez García, R., Hernández Barrera, V., et al. (2009). "Significant differences in the use of healthcare resources of native-born and foreign born in Spain". *BMC Public Health*, 9, 201-213.

Corbacho, C. (2011). "Programa medicación y multiculturalidad". *Universidad Autónoma de Madrid*. 15 junio 2012.

Corsellis, A. (2002). "Formación de los proveedores de servicios públicos para trabajar con intérpretes y traductores. Habilidades y competencias interculturales". In Valero-Garcés, C. (Ed.) *Traducción e Interpretación en los Servicios Públicos. Contextualización, Actualidad y Futuro*. Granada: Comares, 71-90.

—. (2009). *Public Service Interpreting. The First Steps.* Basingstoke, Hampshire: Palgrave Textbooks in Translating and Interpreting. http://us.macmillan.com/series/PalgraveTextbooksinTranslatingandInterpreting [Last accessed April 30th, 2014].

Dodd, C. (1991). *Dynamics of intercultural communication*. Dubuque, IA: W.C. Brown Publishers.

El Mundo. (2003). "Los médicos no entienden a los inmigrantes". *Elmundosalud.com*. http://www.elmundo.es/elmundosalud/2003/01/08/medicina/1042029513.html [Last accessed April 30th, 2014].

Flores G., Abreu M., Barone CP., Bachur R. and Lin H. (2012). "Errors of medical interpretation and their potential clinical consequences: a comparison of professional versus *ad hoc* versus no interpreters". *Annals of Emergency Medicine,* 60(5): 545-53.

Flores, G., Laws, M., Mayo, S., Zuckerman, B., Abreu M., Medina, L. and Hardt, E. (2003). "Errors in medical interpretation and their potential clinical consequences in pediatric encounters". *Pediatrics*, 111(1), 6.

Fustel Fuentes, R. (2009-2010). "Análisis de las traducciones de materiales especializados en el ámbito sanitario en los servicios públicos". 51. Alcalá de Henares

Hamelink, C. (1998). "Human rights: the implementation gap". *Journal of International Communication*, 5, 54-74.

Krewatch, A. (2012). *Two sides of the same coin: the perspective of English speaking patients and doctors in Madrid*. [Unpublished Master's Thesis]. Universidad de Alcalá, Madrid, Spain.

Misra-Herbert, A., MD (2003). "Physician cultural competence: cross-cultural communication improves care". *Cleveland Clinic Journal of Medicine,* 70, 293, 296.

Naranjo, C. (2009). "Cierra el servicio de mediación intercultural". *Madridiario.* 15 junio 2012. http://www.madridiario.es/2009/Enero/canal-social/124912/semsi-cierre-ayuntamiento-denuncia-psoe-zerolo-inmigracion-mediadores-dinamizadores-cear.html [Last accessed April 30th, 2014].

Narayanan, A. (2012) "Interpreters may help shorten hospital stays". *Chicago Tribune*. 18 junio 2012. http://articles.chicagotribune.com/2012-05-25/lifestyle/sns-rt-us-hospital-interpretersbre84o0z4-20120525_1_interpreters-patients-general-internal-medicine [Last accessed April 30th, 2014].

Terraza Núñez, R., Vargas Lorenzo, I., Rodríguez Arjona D., Lizana Alcazo, T. and Vázquez Navarrete, M. (2010). "Políticas sanitarias de ámbito estatal y autonómico para la población inmigrante en España." *Gaceta Sanitaria*, 24, 115-117.

Traber, M. (2008). "Communication is inscribed in human nature". *World Association for Christian Communication.* June 8th, 2012.

U.S. Bureau of Labor Statistics. (2010). "Pharmacist" *U.S. Department of Labor*. May 31st, 2012.

UniversalDoctor. (2011). "Universal Doctor and Tools". http://www.universaldoctor.com/sect/en_GB/9002/Products.html [Last accessed April 30th, 2014].

Valero-Garcés, C. (2001a). "El mediador interlingüístico en los servicios públicos: ¿nuevos principios éticos para nuevas realidades?" *Últimas Corrientes Teóricas en los Estudios de Traducción*. Salamanca: Servicio de Publicaciones de la Universidad, 819-829.

—. (2010). "Challenging communication in doctor / non-native patient encounters. Two perspectives, three types of interaction and some proposals." *The Journal of Specialised Translation*, 14, 230-242.

Williams S., Weinman J. and Dale J. (1998). "Doctor-patient communication and patient satisfaction: a review". *Family Practice*, 15, 480-492.

Women's Clinic & Family Counseling Center. (2006-2010). "Routine gynecological exams." http://www.womens-clinic.org/routine_gynecological_exams.php [Last accessed April 30th, 2014].

CHAPTER FOUR

ENGLISH AS A *LINGUA FRANCA*: A RESOURCE FOR COMMUNICATION IN MULTILINGUAL MEDICAL APPOINTMENTS

Key Points

- English as *lingua franca* and third language as a communication resource in medical appointments.
- The role of cultural differences and its effect on healthcare.
- The effectiveness and quality of written materials in English.
- English-speaking patients' Spanish level and how it affects intercultural communication.

Key Readings

Dodd, C. (1991). *Dynamics of intercultural communication*. Dubuque, IA: W.C. Brown Publishers.

Carrasco Garrido P., Jiménez García R., Hernández Barrera Vl. (2009). "Significant differences in the use of healthcare resources of native-born and foreign born in Spain". *BMC Public Health*, 9, 201–13.

Flores, G., Laws, M., Mayo, S., Zuckerman, B., Abreu M., Medina, L., Hardt, E. (2003). "Errors in medical interpretation and their potential clinical consequences in pediatric encounters". *Pediatrics*, 111, 6.

Misra-Herbert, A., MD (2003). "Physician cultural competence: cross-cultural communication improves care". *Cleveland Clinic Journal of Medicine,* 70, 293, 296.

Valero-Garcés, C. (2010). "Challenging communication in doctor / non-native patient encounters. Two perspectives, three types of interaction and some proposals". *The Journal of Specialised Translation*, 14.

4.1 Introduction

This chapter is an extension of Chapter 3 in so much as it focuses on the use of the English language as a bridge to communicating with foreign patients in the healthcare clinics and institutions of Spain. The study presents data on the different resources used, their type, quality and utility, as well as the results from a survey in which NSSPs rate these resources and the contribution they make to the movement towards multicultural societies in which intercultural communication is a necessity.

4.2 The use of oral English as a communication resource in medical appointments

Following Krewatch's (2012) study, the English-speaking survey participants (ESSPs) were asked if the healthcare specialists that they have seen in Madrid have ever spoken to them in English as a means of communication. The choices that they were given were: "always", "sometimes" and "never". The results show that out of those who have used the healthcare facilities (121 people), only one person (1%) chose "always", indicating that all of the specialists he or she has seen have spoken in English as a means of communication during the appointment. 40 people (approximately 33%) indicated that the specialists they have seen only sometimes have spoken to them in English. Finally, the 80 people (66%) indicated that the specialists that they have seen have never spoken to them in English. Next to the question "Did the healthcare specialists speak to you in English", one ESSP that chose "never" added that the doctors spoke "Very little [English], like 'Hello. How are you" (Comment 1)? When asked "In general, how would you rate the communication level between you and the healthcare specialists you have seen from 1 to 5? (1-little or no communication, 5-fluid communication)" the same person marked the number 3, but below explained "In English 1, In Spanish 4" (Comment 1).

Immediately following the question about how often the healthcare specialists had spoken in English was another about how this affected communication. The ESSPs were asked to choose between: "helped a lot", "helped some", "didn't help" and "made it worse". The person who wrote Comment 1, which indicated that the healthcare specialists in Madrid have always spoken in English seemed very satisfied with doctors. When asked how the doctors' oral English affected communication, this ESSP chose the answer 'helped a lot'. This person also answered 'yes' to the question "Have you ever been offered any written materials in English?". At the end of the survey the level of communication from 1 to 5 (1 meaning little or no communication and 5 meaning fluid communication) a rating of 5 was given.

Of the 41 individuals that said that their specialists either spoke to them in English "sometimes" or "always", 14 people (34%) indicated that this helped a lot, 18 people (44 %) indicated that it helped some, 6 people (15%) indicated that it did not help and 3 people (7%) indicated that it made the situation worse. These results can be considered as good news for the specialists that have used English to communicate with their patients. If those who chose "helped some" and "helped a lot" are combined, then that suggests that 32 people (78%) of the ESSPs believe that when their doctors speak to them in English it affects communication in a positive way. Those who chose "didn't help" simply suggest that the specialists who spoke in English neither affected communication positively nor negatively. This leaves only 7% who in choosing "made it worse" suggest that communication was affected negatively when spoken to in English.

The results from the survey regarding healthcare specialists that use English as a communication resource lead to the conclusion that there are still doctors in Madrid that either do not know sufficient English for use in a medical setting or chose not to use it for other reasons. This is unfortunate because the majority (78%) of English-speaking patients who are treated by doctors that do speak to them in English have reported that they have benefited from it.

Box 4.1.

Comment 1

In an interview conducted in Spanish, a radiologist at the Hospital Reina Sofia in Cordoba, Spain, was asked the following: "*How would you rate the level of English of Spanish physicians in comparison with that of your colleagues in other countries*?"

His answer was: *Interestingly enough, medical English is quite easy for the Spanish and the French, given that 50% of the terminology is of Greek and Latin origin and is therefore well-understood. However, we have difficulty pronouncing anything that is easily read, such as edema, for example. Despite the advantage that comes with knowing a romance language, we let the opportunity go to waste to the extent that a person from Japan can reach the same level in just 5 years. Generally, the rest of Europe enjoys a more advanced level in the language than we do.* (Tardón, 2012) (My own translation).

The response given by this doctor is consistent with Comment 2 (below): This information suggests that it is possible that the reason that healthcare specialists do not choose to speak in English with English-speaking patients is due to their incapability of orally expressing themselves in the language. In this instance the ESSP indicated a level 5 of Spanish on a scale from 1 to 5 (1 meaning beginner level and 5 meaning fluent level). This high level of Spanish was probably what made the patient dismiss the doctor's attempts to speak in English with what appears to be a lower level. If the doctor had been able to pronounce medical terms correctly in English perhaps they would not have had to revert to Spanish in order to carry on with the appointment.

Box 4.2.

Comment 2: *Some doctors have tried to speak to me in English, but usually I ask them to switch back to Spanish. Most medical terminology is derived from Latin so I actually understood them better with their Spanish pronunciation than when they tried to explain things to me in English.*

Comment 3 is a statement regarding the English level of Madrid doctors that was taken from an ESSP. This comment includes both positive and negative aspects. On one hand, the ESSP praises the care and expertise of Madrid healthcare specialists while on the other hand criticizes the availability of those who speak English. Although being friendly and experienced are good qualities to have, they do not address the doctors' ability to communicate well with the patient. Unfortunately, the downside to the comment is what directly relates to the possibility of an English-speaking patient being able to communicate with a Madrid doctor through speaking in English.

Box 4.3.

Comment 3: *I can speak for the healthcare specialists who had me as a patient, and say that they were excellent professionals and the level of care and expertise was very high. But if I didn't have the level of Spanish I do, I would assume the feedback would be very negative, because in my experience very few healthcare professionals speak English, let alone enough to describe complex issues related to your health.*

Another important point made in the statement is that health issues by nature tend to be very complex. This leaves no room for doctors to have a poor level of English if they are planning on using it as the sole resource to interact with patients. This is due to the fact that medical information given correctly may be the difference between life and death; in other words, a misunderstanding between the doctor and patient has the potential of having fatal consequences. Therefore, Comment 4 may not always be comforting news, unless of course there was a way to be sure that the doctor in question is proficient in medical English. In this sense it is fitting to add that even native English-speakers who have not studied medicine are most likely not proficient in medical English.

Box 4.4.

Comment 4: *I find most doctors very eager to practice their English.*

On a lighter note, not all comments made by the ESSPs regarding English being spoken by healthcare specialists were negative. Comment 5, for example, suggests that in Madrid there are doctors who are able to communicate effectively with English-speaking patients using various resources including oral English.

Box 4.5.

Comment 5: *In general, I have been extremely impressed with healthcare in Madrid. Even from the very beginning, barely able to speak the language (I had my dictionary) there has been a great effort to make sure I was calm and knew what was happening. They have always spoken slowly and clearly, used what little (or significant) level of English they had. Excellent nonverbal communication!*

4.3 The role of cultural differences and its effect on healthcare

One issue which proved to be a common concern among those who shared their thoughts is the cultural barrier that they have experienced between themselves and the doctors that they have seen in Madrid. Approximately 73% of the ESSPs who added personal comments originate from the United States, yet only 57% of those who participated in the survey (including those who did not include a personal comment) are from the United States. This suggests that Americans are more likely to have specific information that they consider important enough to share. Interestingly enough, 100% of those who in their comments alluded to cultural problems being the root of non-communication were of American origin. This indicates that there may be greater cultural differences between Americans and Spaniards with respect to healthcare compared to those that exist between the Spanish and people from the UK, Canada and Ireland.

In Comment 6, one ESSP actually went as far as to say that the root of the communication problem that exists between doctors and patients is due to differences in culture while language is simply a secondary issue that just adds to the complication. This is an example of a situation where a problem was created because from the beginning there was a negative atmosphere stemming from the awkward situation. In this case the patient and the doctor are unknowingly relying on two different social norms.

Box 4.6.

Comment 6: *I've found more of a cultural than language barrier. In the US I am used to the doctor asking questions, while here the patient is expected to talk and tell what the problem is. This system is much more difficult for someone with limited language proficiency.*

David Lewis defines social norms as "customary rules of behavior that coordinate our interactions with others. Once a particular way of doing things becomes established as a rule, it continues in force because we prefer to conform to the rule given the expectation that others are going to conform" (Lewis, 1969 as cited in Young, 2007). In the aforementioned example the American patient assumes that the doctor will be the conversation starter and will ask what is necessary to obtain the information needed to come to the right diagnosis. On the other hand, the doctor assumes that the patient will come prepared to give a speech providing the doctor with all of the information that he or she needs to reach the same end. In the first scenario, the patient takes on a passive role while the doctor takes command, but in the second scenario the doctor is the one who takes on the passive role. When these opposing methods collide, this could lead to an initial silence. Neither person would know who should start the conversation due to the conflicting social norms that each are accustomed to.

Comment 7 was taken from another ESSP who supports the theory that cultural differences led to confusion and that the language barrier further complicates matters. This person gives a specific example of what Americans expect based on their previous experiences with doctors in the United States. A typical eye doctor check-up is used to portray how most are accustomed to a step-by-step explanation of everything that is going to occur throughout the appointment. This comment does not suggest that there are no doctors in Madrid that give their patients this type of attention; rather that it is fairly common to be less communicative. The cultural situation mentioned is dangerous because the patient may not know that he or she needs to be more assertive to get all of the important information. Also, due to not being accustomed to asking for this information, the patient might feel nervous or even too embarrassed to ask for it. Lack of communication may lead to loss of pertinent details which may or may not have a negative effect on the patient. In this case, the quality of the healthcare would be compromised.

Box 4.7.

***Comment** 7: I think my communication issues with healthcare professionals in Madrid stemmed not so much from the language barrier as from differing expectations about what needed to be communicated. For example, doctors in the US usually give you a general overview about your appointment when you first sit down with them: 'Today we're going to do some tests to make sure you don't have glaucoma or cataracts, and then we're going to check your vision to see if your prescription has changed.' And they definitely warn you before starting any procedures: 'Now we're going to do the glaucoma test. You're going to feel a puff of air in each eye--it's important to keep your head still.' Doctors in Madrid do not necessarily communicate in either of these categories--they may prep the patient and/or explain the procedure, or they may just start drawing blood (or whatever) without any warning or explanation. I think it can be a shift for Anglo patients to realize they really have to be their own advocate in the Spanish health system and not to be afraid to demand information from their doctors -- it's not necessarily a given that you'll receive any otherwise.*

This comment is consistent with the results from a study conducted in the United Kingdom about doctor-patient communication and patient satisfaction (Williams, Weinman, Dale 1998). Data comes from a sample of 150 patients who were attending 1 of 15 physicians in a general medicine out-patient clinic. An observer coded the physicians' behavior with a 30-item checklist developed for the study. Patients completed a 23-

item satisfaction questionnaire. The results indicated that patient satisfaction is highly correlated with information-giving by the doctor.

The results taken from the above study indicate that British people as well as Americans value thorough appointments in which they receive information and advice from their physicians. These results provide a logical explanation for the reasons why some English-speaking residents of Madrid chose to make the following statements (Comments 8-10) that denote an unsatisfied tone:

Box 4.8.

Comment 8: *Communication in the Spanish healthcare system is limited, no matter what languages you speak.*

Box 4.9.

Comment 9: *In general, I find that healthcare specialists here are less communicative than what an American is used to. They don't ask as many questions or give as many explanations, and seem a little annoyed when you ask lots of clarifying questions.*

Box 4.10.

Comment 10: *I never really felt like Spanish doctors will sit down and talk to you, and that they are often dismissive – but I'm not sure if it comes from a miscommunication or a cultural thing.*

Information becoming "lost in translation" is not the only risk that comes from the lack of a mutual understanding of social norms. There is also the chance of false assumptions which have the potential of effecting healthcare quality. Comment 11 was also taken from an American ESSP and is used to exemplify this notion. There are several ways of interpreting how the patient felt and what led him or her to such conclusions. One way is to agree in assuming that since the doctor did not give the patient the care that he or she expected, this must mean that the doctor lacks compassion. The fact is that there are many reasons that the patient could have perceived the doctor as uncompassionate. However, when taking into consideration the accounts from other Americans that suggest that culture is the source of miscommunication with Spanish doctors; one theory may be that the patient was simply unaware of Spanish healthcare norms.

Assuming this is true, the patient most likely confused typical doctor behavior with being rude and apathetic.

Box 4.11.

Comment 11: *The doctors don't give the necessary care expected. They don't have much compassion.*

Whether or not the patient made an accurate assumption is not the most important issue. If the goal is to achieve a full understanding between the doctor and the patient, false assumptions may become an obstacle that can interrupt and nullify the entire communication process. In the article mentioned above, Williams et al. state that:

The expression of negative affect has been shown to be negatively related to patient satisfaction. Inui and colleagues found that tension in the tone of either the doctor or patient was negatively related to satisfaction. Patient anxiety-nervousness was also negatively related to patient satisfaction (Williams, Weinman, Dale 1998).

The quality of the healthcare received could be altered due to the patient's negative perception of the doctor's behavior. For instance, when feeling uncomfortable, the patient may conclude that the doctor is inadequate and disregard any sort of advice or diagnosis given. Moreover, the patient may choose not to share relevant medical details such as symptoms, as a result of feeling inhibited. Rather than communication being promoted, it would actually be discouraged, which defeats the purpose.

The next example given by Krewatch (2012) is taken from Vorvick and Storck (2012) to illustrate the communicative difficulty due to culture is based on a specific appointment between a Spanish gynecologist and an American patient. All women, regardless of cultural background, are urged to visit the gynecologist regularly for a Pap smear. According to the National Institutes of Health, starting at age 21 women should have a Pap smear every two years. This routine check-up includes the collection of a sample of a woman's cervical cells which afterwards are sent to a laboratory to be tested for cancer or abnormalities. Although this test is performed both in Spain and English-speaking countries, the appointment is not necessarily done in the same manner. The following is a quote (Comment 12) taken from one of the surveys that shows how an American's expectation of how the appointment should go had an effect on communication.

Box 4.12.

Comment 12: *I do remember one specific time when I had to go to the doctor back in my first year that I was living in Madrid. I went to the gynecologist and I thought I understood what the nurse wanted me to do (she never spoke to me in English and I never did request that she speak in English). I was baffled at why I was told to wait in the waiting area for a good 45 minutes even though part of my appointment had already taken place. Then the nurse came back and asked me if I had to go to the bathroom. I replied with some sort of 'nah I'm good' kind of attitude and she looked surprised. Here I didn't realize that she was waiting for my bladder to fill up so she could do an ultrasound. At the time I didn't even realize that she had said the word 'vejiga' [bladder] or I would have asked her to define it or clarify what she was saying. I only thought she was asking me to wait in the waiting room for a little while...*

The possibility that in Spain a Pap smear may be followed by a vaginal ultrasound was not something that the patient had previously considered, most likely because in her country of origin she had never had a similar gynecological appointment. In the United States ultrasounds are not part of the routine gynecological exam. Below is a six-step explanation given by a clinic in California of how gynecological exams are performed:

1. First you'll need to undress and put on a cover. When you lie on the exam table, you will have a sheet to cover your legs.
2. Your clinician will check your breasts for any lumps or changes that may lead to cancer. Be sure to ask about checking your breasts at home.
3. Your clinician will check the outside of your vagina. Then the clinician will gently open the vagina with a speculum.
4. Your clinician will take a few cells from your cervix for the Pap test. You may feel a pinch or a cramp, but it only takes a few seconds.
5. Next your clinician will perform a pelvic exam - a check of your sex organs by placing two fingers in your vagina while gently pressing on your stomach. If it is hard to feel your organs this way, your clinician may also place a finger in your rectum. This can make you feel like you have to go to the bathroom.
6. Tell the clinician if you have had any rashes, bumps, pain or discharge. You may need other tests. (*Women's Clinic & Family Counseling Center*, 2006-2010).

Step number five is especially important because there lies the difference between the exam that the survey ESSP described in Madrid compared to exams performed in the United States. Instead of including an ultrasound, a tactile pelvic exam is done.

As Krewatch (2012) points out, the most obvious cause of the problem that arose when the American patient was told to wait in the waiting room until she felt the need to urinate is the language barrier. If only the patient and the gynecologist had been able to communicate in the same language or through an interpreter, maybe the miscommunication could have been avoided. However, there exists a possible solution to the language problem; common social norms. If the doctor and patient had in fact come from cultures that practice the same routine gynecological procedure, the language barrier would not have been as likely to lead to misunderstandings. This is evidence that understanding cultural differences is essential for true communication to occur.

4.4 Pre-appointment preparation and written materials in English

In addition to assessing the frequency with which spoken English is used as a tool for communication between English-speaking patients and Madrid healthcare specialists, another survey objective was to determine how often written materials in English are used. Written materials refer to any medical information or documents such as pamphlets or patient forms. Graph 4.1 represents the results from the question "Have you ever been offered any written materials in English at a health visit?" As shown in Graph 4.1, approximately 97% of the ESSPs that have visited healthcare facilities while residing in Madrid reported that they have not been offered while 3% reported that they had. These results were quite surprising considering that the *Dirección General de Atención Primaria del Servicio Madrileño de Salud* issues health publications in English. As this is a public body, the health-related materials that are printed are intended for public health facilities. Because the vast majority of ESSPs indicated that they have not been offered written materials in English, this may suggest that their health visits have been in private facilities where these materials are not available.

Based on several ESSP comments, it is clear that certain patients feel most comfortable using written materials to aid communication. Comments 13-15 taken from the survey are examples of patients who chose to prepare for doctor's visits by translating words or sentences they thought to be of importance from Spanish to English before-hand. All of them were written by ESSPs who indicated that they had never been offered written materials in English while at doctor's appointments in Madrid.

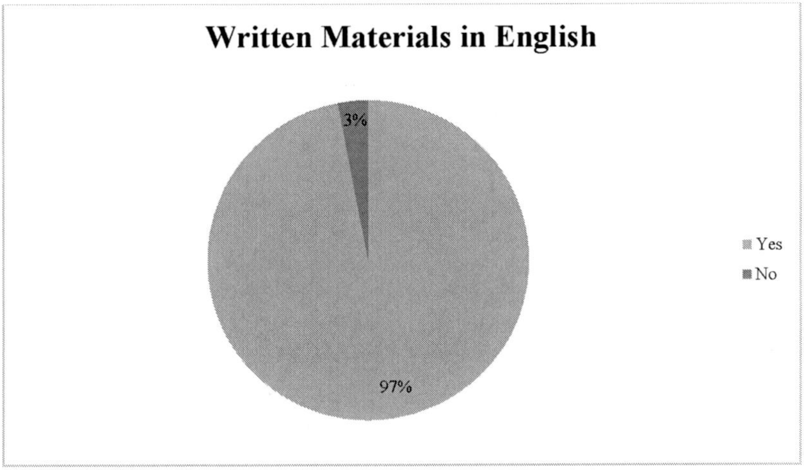

Graph 4.1: Percentage of ESSPs offered written materials in English while at health visits

Comment 13 comes from someone whose Spanish level was rated as 3. This may be the reason for feeling the need to try additional communication methods, rather than simply relying on speaking in Spanish. Instead, this person took the liberty of becoming familiarized with vocabulary in Spanish that may be useful when speaking to doctors. The effort made, however, did not seem to be enough based on the remark expressing concern about possibly missing something. Whether or not this person could have benefited from materials in writing about pertinent medical information is unknown, but it is possible that he or she would have felt less uneasy about missing something if it was all on paper; able to be consulted at any time.

Box 4.13.

Comment 13: *I have always looked up any important words or health specific words before a visit to the doctors. Though I generally feel confident in my understanding of the doctor, but I always feel nervous that I have missed something.*

The person who wrote Comment 14 indicated a rating of 5 regarding Spanish level. In this case it is conceivable that speaking in Spanish may be the only means of communication necessary. Nevertheless, this person considered it necessary to come to doctor's appointments prepared. The fact that these occurrences took place during the earlier years in Madrid suggests that maybe the Spanish level was lower which led to the need to look into different options. In this comment it is also pointed out that the person has no experience going to public healthcare facilities which may account for never being offered written materials in English. One positive aspect is never feeling discriminated against for being from a different country which could otherwise have an effect on communication. This ESSP chose to offer the doctor relevant written information to aid understanding during the health visit which suggests that he or she may have benefited from receiving the same.

Box 4.14.

Comment 14: *I find that most doctors and nurses make an effort to be understood (at least in private health care, I've had no personal experience in the public system). I've never felt like I was treated any differently because I wasn't from Spain. Admittedly, my first years here were a lot tougher, and I sometimes consulted a dictionary and wrote down words on a paper to help explain myself better. I also always asked to have things clearly written in Spanish so that I would be able to understand things easily.*

Comment 15 comes from a person who had a Spanish language rating of 2. Being that this rating corresponds to an elementary level, it probably created the need to prepare something in Spanish before going to the doctor. This case is slightly different in that the patient chose to use a machine translator, namely Google Translate.

According to Jacob (2012), recently, one of Google's research scientists, Ashish Venugopal, spoke to local media about the programme and how it works. In a video conference from the Google Campus in California, Ashish explained why translation errors happen. 'It all boils down to data,' he said. 'The programme works so well that it doesn't realise when there is a mistake. We try to imbue the system with statistical knowledge of the language, but we can't do all of it, so there are errors sometimes. It's important to keep in perspective what the role of Google Translate is,' Ashish said. 'It's not to take over the job of professional translators. The programme can never capture emotion or translate speech in a beautiful way, but it can tell you what is being said'.

Box 4.15.

Comment 15: *Whenever there was a situation that required a doctor's visit I always wrote down what was wrong and what I needed to say and translated it via Google Translate. Afterwards, I would have either a coworker or a flatmate reread the translation and make sure everything was grammatically correct and made sense. Then off to the doctor I went. Sometimes I did get a doctor that spoke English, other times I didn't and they would write down what was wrong (the diagnosis more or less) and I would translate it later. There was one office that I frequented where the secretaries spoke English. The doctors that did speak English were 30 or younger. Possibly still in med school or post grad.*

Based on the information given by Ashish Venugopal, people who use Google Translate run the risk of having translation errors. Many paper dictionaries provide contexts and various possible translations to choose from, whereas machine translators such as Google Translate are forced to render only one translation for each word. This may not be of importance when translating something that does not require a precise translation. Health-related issues, however, have a tendency of being quite complicated and detailed. Therefore, medical translation errors may lead to an undesirable outcome for the patient such as an incorrect diagnosis.

As for the English speaking patients (ESSPs), Comments 13-15 demonstrate that it took some time to plan how they were going to communicate with their respective doctors by using dictionaries and machine translators as an aid in writing notes. This demonstrates initiative taken on their part to make for a successful doctor's appointment. On the other hand, survey results indicate that nearly none of the Madrid healthcare centers offers written material in English to better accommodate their English-speaking patients.

4.5 (Deficient) Quality in resources (and some) consequences

Some of the ESSPs who included comments in their surveys give the impression that they are unaware of the dangers of their healthcare specialists using certain resources as means for communication. In fact, they confuse these tactics as being quite helpful, when in reality they can have a rather damaging effect. The tendency, then, is to naively praise the specialists for a job well done, rather than realizing the unprofessionalism involved in using such resources. These tactics include: the use of internet translation, nonverbal communication and *ad hoc* interpreters. Comment 16 provides an ideal example of an ESSP who found it especially kind of her doctor to use the internet to facilitate communication.

Box 4.16.

Comment 16: *The woman doctor I saw went to her computer to use the internet to translate a word I said in English to Spanish (while speaking in Spanish) to better understand what we were talking about. It was very kind of her. I really appreciated it.*

It is impossible to know exactly what website or program the doctor was using and how reliable the source was, however based on the aforementioned information about Google Translate, it can be concluded that a doctor using a low-cost literal translation from the internet would be just as risky.

According to Misra-Herbert, a doctor from the Department of General Internal Medicine at Cleveland Clinic, "gestures are not universal, and their use may cause unnecessary miscommunication" (Misra-Herbert, 2003). This is precisely the reason that one cannot assume that messages sent through nonverbal communication are always going to be clear regardless of what culture a person comes from. Sometimes one gesture may mean two completely different things to two people from different cultures. In addition, certain gestures may only exist in one culture leaving people from other cultures bewildered wondering what it could possibly mean. This uncertainty creates a larger margin for serious errors in healthcare settings. In Comment 17, as well as in Comment 4 found above, the ESSPs believe that nonverbal communication is the solution to the problems caused by the language barrier.

The final dangerous resource addressed here is *ad hoc* interpreters. The results from the survey for the English-speakers show that using any type of interpreter, trained or untrained, was not common. Only 11.5% of all healthcare visitors reported having done so. The most shocking evidence though, was the fact that none of those who had used an interpreter in a health visit had used a professional interpreter, meaning that all of them could be classified as *ad hoc*; the majority being friends and family members. Comment 18 is from a girl who chose to use a family member as her interpreter, and Comment 19 is from a person who served as an interpreter for a friend.

Box 4.17.

> ***Comment 17:*** *I found it difficult to explain my condition at the time because I've not studied medical Spanish. I couldn't fully elaborate! Going to the same doctor both times made it easier because I think he was very patient with me and understood that I'm not a native Spanish speaker. I tried explaining my family's medical history, and although I wasn't sure how to say some terms, he worked with [me] and used gestures to aid communication.*

Box 4.18.

> ***Comment 18:*** *I gave birth to my daughter in 2009 in a Spanish hospital. During labor my husband (who is Spanish) would act as an interpreter between me and the doctors. It's difficult not always being able to advocate for myself. I did have a doctor during my pregnancy who spoke English very well and it was great to be able to understand everything! In my experience I have had several doctors ask me if I preferred them to speak English.*

Box 4.19.

> ***Comment 19:*** *Although I have never used an interpreter I did act as an interpreter for an American friend (female 26 [years old]) who did not speak any Spanish. The health care provider spoke little to no English and had I not acted as interpreter my friend would not have been able to communicate. She was not offered any materials in English.*

In a study carried out by Flores, Abreu, Barone, Bachur and Lin whose purpose was to compare interpreter errors and their potential consequences in encounters with professional versus *ad hoc* versus no interpreters. The results were as follows: "Compared with professional interpreters, *ad hoc* interpreters and having no interpreters resulted in significantly higher proportions of omissions and false-fluency errors" (Flores, Abreu, Barone, Bachur, Lin, 2012).

Ad hoc interpreters tend to complicate communication based on a sense of inhibition either felt by the patient, the interpreter or both. This inhibition stems from a previously established relationship made between the patient and the interpreter. Depending on the reason for the health visit, the patient may feel embarrassed about sharing certain information, or the interpreter may feel uncomfortable with interpreting sensitive matters because of being influenced by emotions. Comment 18 is an example of how both patient and interpreter would be affected by any bad news about the baby which may affect the quality of the interpretation. It is also possible that the patient may not want to share personal feminine information with her husband present. A professional Spanish language interpreter at Stanford (California) University Medical Center, Linda Haffner, shared a relevant personal story about a family member (child) being used as an interpreter for her Latin-American mother:

The call is to help with a pregnant woman who may have a still birth. As I enter the patient's room, the first thing I see is a beautiful girl with haunting big brown eyes-the patient's 7-year-old daughter. I introduce myself with the proper Spanish salutation. The mother seems upset, but the daughter looks very distressed and frightened. The child is shaking and with a quiet voice says to me 'No podía explicarle a mi mama todo lo que los doctores me decían' ('I couldn't explain to my mom everything the doctors were telling me.'). I quickly discovered that this little girl was used as the interpreter during the ultrasound examination and was told to tell her mother (her little brother-to-be) is dead. This revelation stuns me. I sit and hold the little girl on my lap, trying to comfort her as she holds me tightly. I softly talk to her about what has happened, and she starts to weep with big, slow tears. To me, one of the saddest moments is when she says to me, in a pleading voice, 'Maybe my little brother's heart will work when he comes out of my mother's stomach' (Haffner 1992).

The problem is that the three communication tactics mentioned above are all cost effective. There is no need to spend money on gestures, *ad hoc* interpreters nor using the internet that is already being paid for. This is what makes such tactics as appealing and popular. Hardly any effort or money is spent compared to hiring a professional interpreter.

In addition to money issues, the awareness of the importance for using trained interpreters is low. People do not realize how important they are, until they are faced with a terrible situation caused by unprofessional translating/interpreting. In the end, the cost, whether emotional or monetary, may end up being much greater due to the errors made by relying on overly literal online translations, ambiguous body language or untrained interpreters.

4.6 Language proficiency and how it effects intercultural communication

It is important to take into account the level of Spanish that the ESSPs have when analyzing the data collected from the surveys because it may influence their perception of the communication level that they had with doctors in medical appointments. The ESSPs were asked to self-evaluate their current Spanish proficiency on a scale from 1 to 5 (1 meaning beginner level and 5 meaning fluent level). A more precise way to analyze this data would be to consider the following key: 1=beginner, 2=elementary, 3=intermediate, 4=advanced, 5=fluent. According to this scale it would be accurate to describe a rating of 3 as equivalent to an intermediate level. The average proficiency level taken from all of the ESSPs was approximately 3.5. This indicates that on average they spoke Spanish at slightly above an intermediate level at the time of completing the survey. However, due to the change in level over time, it is impossible to know each person's level at the time of all of the medical appointments that they went to which is why the current level is used as a reference.

The ESSPs were also asked to evaluate the general level of communication that they believe to have had with Madrid healthcare specialists on a scale from 1 to 5 (This question only applied to those who had used healthcare facilities (1 meaning little or no communication and 5 meaning fluid communication). On average the ESSPs felt that their communication level was equivalent to a 3.7 rating. In order to better interpret what this rating means in terms of communication the following key shall be used: 1=poor, 2=fair, 3=good, 4=very good, 5=excellent. This means that the 3.7 rating corresponds to a good/quite good communication. However, due to their relatively high level of Spanish, it is possible that the ESSPs perceived their communication level with the doctors to be higher than they would have if they had no knowledge of the Spanish language. Therefore, whether this rating is based on the resources used by the doctor or the patients' ability to speak in Spanish with their physicians cannot be determined. In an attempt to solve this problem, the personal accounts of the ESSPs which provide additional information have been used as a guide in finding explanations for the data.

As previously stated, 66% of the ESSPs indicated that the healthcare specialists that they have visited in Madrid have never spoken to them in English. The most obvious assumption is the reason that the doctors chose not to speak in English to native English speakers is that they must not have known English at all or not well enough to use it as a resource in a medical setting. Another explanation is that they simply did not want to talk in English either out of embarrassment or stubbornness. Although the tendency is to wonder what is wrong with the doctor, it is necessary to take both parties into account. When doing so this leads to another explanation that does not place the blame on the doctor, rather on the patient. This is when it becomes clear that the patients' level of Spanish can definitely have an effect on whether or not English is spoken at all during the visits. With regard to the survey question "Did the healthcare specialists speak to you in English?" one ESSP answered N/A [Not applicable], and added "I didn't need them to" **(Comment 20).**

The next two quotes are taken from ESSPs who expressed similar information that has affected the communication level with their doctors. Comment 21 was taken from a person who rated his/her Spanish level as 5 (fluent) and the communication level with doctors as 4 (quite good). Comment 22 was taken from a person who rated his/her Spanish level as 4 (advanced) and communication level with doctors as 3 (good).

Box 4.20.

Comment 21: *Since I've been living here for 4 years and I feel that I am fluent in Spanish I really haven't had many problems in explaining what I need or understanding what doctors say to me.*

Box 4.21.

Comment 22: *Since I have been living in Madrid since I was 18, my Spanish level has gone from very low to quite high.*

A large amount of ESSPs originate from the US which is a country that has a very diverse population. As reported in the 2010 census brief issued by the United States Census Bureau, there is no official language in the US, English is the most common language spoken while Spanish is the second (Ennis, Ríos-Vargas, Albert, 2011). In the census brief the term "Hispanic or Latino" was used to refer to a person of Cuban, Mexican, Puerto Rican, South or Central American, or other Spanish culture or origin regardless of race. According to the 2010 Census,

308.7 million people resided in the United States on April 1, 2010, of which 50.5 million (or 16%) were of Hispanic or Latino origin. The Hispanic population increased from 35.3 million in 2000 when this group made up 13 percent of the total population. Between 2000 and 2010, the Hispanic population grew by 43 percent, which was four times the growth in the total population at 10 percent (Ennis, Ríos-Vargas, Albert 2011).

The information taken from the census indicates that a significant group of American citizens originate from Spanish-speaking countries. It is therefore possible that some of the ESSPs also come from "Hispanic or Latino" backgrounds and are more likely to have already been bilingual in English and Spanish before arriving in Spain. This may be part of the reason that the Spanish proficiency level average of 3.5 and not lower.

Comment 23 was taken from a bilingual American ESSP:

Box 4.22.

> ***Comment 23:*** *I'm of Costa Rican origin. I was born, raised and educated in the US and my mother spoke to me in Spanish and my father in English, so I've always addressed the healthcare professionals in Spain in Spanish. If I ever needed to say a word/medical term in English I pretty much just got a blank face as a response.*

This person unsurprisingly gave a rating of 5 for the communication level with the physician. Thanks to the comment that was written on the survey, an external factor was accounted for as an explanation for such a high rating of the communication level. It is, however, uncertain the number of survey participants that were in similar situations.

The previous survey statements together with the average Spanish level of 3.5 are evidence of the great possibility that English-speaking residents in Madrid have been educated in the Spanish language. While this may be part of the reason that so many Madrid doctors do not need to speak to their patients in English, it also may account for such a high rating (3.7) of the level of communication that the ESSPs had with their doctors. This means that before assuming that a good/quite good communication level was achieved by the resources and techniques employed by the healthcare specialists, one must consider that it may be attributed to English-speaking patients' ability to adapt to their doctors' mother tongue. This presents the troubling notion that the communication level rating may be dependent solely upon patient Spanish proficiency. Graph 4.2 describes the correlation between communication level (dependent variable) and the Spanish level of the ESSP (independent variable).

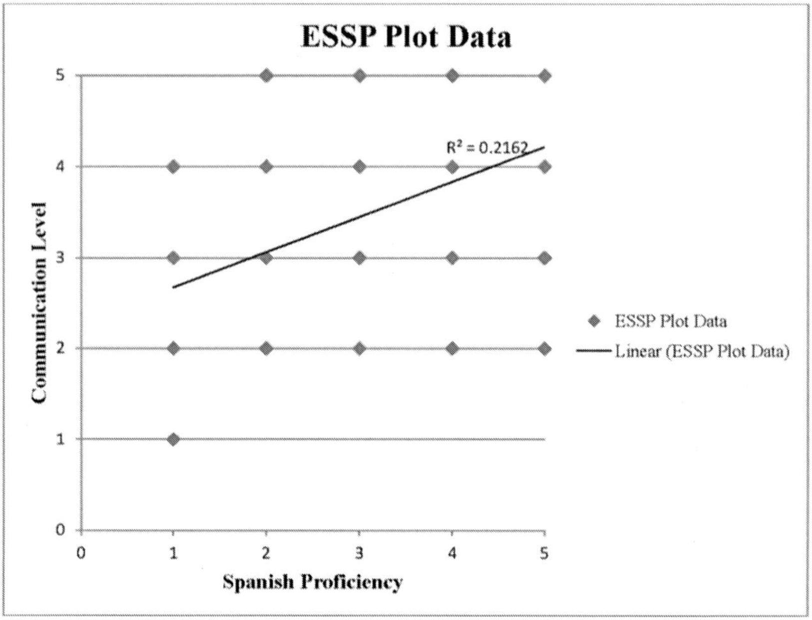

Graph 4.2: Scatter plot displaying the dependency level of ESSP communication on ESSP Spanish proficiency

The correlation coefficient value (on a scale of -1.0 to 1.0) of this graph is approximately 0.46 which means that the correlation between communication level between Madrid healthcare specialists and ESSPs is moderately positive. When squaring this number the result is 0.21 which indicates that in roughly 21% of the cases as Spanish proficiency goes up, so does the rating that the ESSPs give to the communication level. Since this only happens in 21% of the cases, it can be concluded that in 79% of the cases (the majority of the time) the communication level rating depends on other variables, such as the resources that doctors use to communicate with their English-speaking patients. This places a significant importance on the doctor's capability of interacting successfully with patients.

In conclusion, although Spanish proficiency may play a role in patient-doctor communication, it is not the only factor. Therefore, average communication level rating of 3.7 (good/quite good) is not solely based on Spanish proficiency which indicates that the majority of English-speaking patients manage to communicate effectively with Madrid doctors by other means. This means that it is possible that the few resources that healthcare specialists are currently using, in spite of being scarce, are effective in communicating with their patients. This information suggests an improvement on specialists' part. Although there is plenty of room to improve further, it seems as though progress is being made and the Madrid healthcare system is taking the initial steps towards accommodating their English-speaking patients. This is positive news which indicates that there is a light at the end of the tunnel.

Below is a list of positive testimonials (Comments 24-27) from ESSPs about their good experiences with healthcare visits in Madrid regarding intercultural communication:

Box 4.23.

Comment 24: *One relatively positive experience I had was with a dermatologist in Madrid. He spoke slowly and clearly and even drew diagrams and pictures to make sure I understood everything correctly. He didn't rush through the appointment and really seemed to care about helping me.*

Box 4.24.

Comment 25: I *had an operation a few years ago, which is a pretty scary thing in any situation, especially in a foreign country with surgeons and doctors and nurses speaking to you in a foreign language during pre-op, surgery, and post op-procedures, but I had a wonderful experience in that I felt very comfortable and well taken care of the whole time; including my four day stay in the hospital after the operation. I have private health care and have always had the pleasure of dealing with professionals who took the time to make sure I understood everything that was going on before proceeding.*

Box 4.25.

Comment 26: *I personally have had very positive experiences here in Spain regarding visits to the doctor. Both physicians I have come into contact with have been very understanding and patient with my Spanish and have been equally as patient when explaining anything to me regarding prescription instructions, recommendations, etc.*

Box 4.26.

Comment 27: *In all my experiences at a healthcare facility, I was very well treated and most doctors made an effort to speak slowly and to make sure I understood everything properly.*

4.7 Conclusions

The research done on this topic, together with the data collected from surveys and interviews in this chapter and in Chapter 3, led to the following final conclusions:

Although action has been taken in an attempt to respond to the needs of all residents of Madrid regardless of cultural background, inequalities still exist for migrants and visitors who do not speak Spanish when it comes to accessing healthcare. Medical specialists in Madrid tend to rely on communication resources such as *ad hoc* interpreters and machine translators, and are reluctant to work with professionals in the field. In many cases official interpretation/translation services are not readily accessible to healthcare professionals. Below, we provide a brief summary of the study presented in previous pages as well as some comments about possible solutions which might lead to a better future for both English-speaking patients and medical staff:

The fact that Spaniards generally possess a low level of English creates certain difficulty for English-speaking patients and, given that English is spoken as a second language by people all over the world, possibly even for patients who are not from countries where English or Spanish is the official language. Nevertheless, the healthcare workers surveyed did indicate that they felt they possessed some knowledge of the language and said that they used it, albeit some more than others, during medical encounters with foreign patients. There are situations in which attempts to communicate in a language in which one has little knowledge can lead to problems and even more confusion. This may be due to difficulties in comprehension, pronunciation or poor use of the language. In those cases in which the doctor, nurse, etc. does not have a high enough command of English, it is advisable not to attempt to communicate in English and to instead seek other solutions such as providing educational materials in English or using a professional interpreter. It would be wise to create a special English test which, if passed by the healthcare worker, would authorize that person to use English as a tool for communicating with patients. Otherwise, the staff member would abstain from speaking in English with patients regardless of his or her knowledge of the language.

4.8 Tips for the future

In the long term, Spain should come up with an effective way to improve the level of English of its citizens. In today's world, English is used as a global language and is fundamental to intercultural communication. The non-English speaking countries having the highest level of English are those which belong to the European Union. However, in spite of the fact that Spain entered the EU in 1986, it continues to lag far behind other key economic powers due to the disadvantage that not having a high level of English poses. Knowing English is not only helpful in the international world of business, but also within one's own country. Many of the healthcare professionals surveyed expressed an interest in improving their English and were also interested in the possibility of having more information available in the language. This indicates that these professionals have already found themselves in situations where it would have been helpful to use English as a resource in communication but where they were not able to do so for whatever reason. The fact that healthcare professionals are aware of how useful it would be to be able to communicate in English at an advanced level is a positive sign because it suggests that they will likely make every effort to be able to do so.

There are several possibilities open when it comes to overcoming linguistic and cultural barriers. One of these would be to restructure healthcare policy as it pertains to the migrant community, making it more ambitious. On a fundamental level, this must include having more information available in foreign languages about the healthcare system, how it works and how to access these services. There should be a wider variety of healthcare pamphlets available, given that migrants and visitors should have information on the same healthcare topics that members of the native community have. This could also include a requirement that anyone planning to become a doctor first take an instructional course in which they would be taught how to treat foreign patients. This way, they would be familiar with the topic beforehand. This would avoid uncomfortable situations in which the doctor gives off the impression of being inexperienced and unprofessional. In order for there to be a policy that works properly, perhaps the most important element is to implement what has been proposed. It is not enough to create a detailed plan that includes solutions to all the problems that arise from difficulties in communication, it is also essential that each proposed plan be executed. For this to occur there must be a way to verify that the plans are being carried out according to the stipulations of the policy.

Another way to improve intercultural communication in healthcare settings would be to make medical professionals aware of and inform them about how dangerous it can be to use certain machine resources or *ad hoc* interpreters. We must refute the idea that it is more costly to provide professional interpreters than to use other resources that are "free". Service providers must realize that the resources that seem so cost-effective are those which lead to more omissions, additions and distortions of the information being transmitted. These errors are the reason that less is accomplished during medical encounters and that the patients must sometimes return more often, which in turn requires more money and creates a more costly situation in the end. Apart from possibly being more cost-efficient, having professional interpreter services could mean higher quality medical consultations. Patients would not feel inhibited in front of family members or acquaintances when speaking about personal topics and the interpretations would be more faithful to the original.

It should also be mentioned that the results of this study do not represent all English-speaking residents or all healthcare professionals in the area. Some elements which may have influenced the study are: limited time to conduct the study and certain difficulty in obtaining special permits in order to conduct surveys and interviews with healthcare professionals. More research, but also cooperation, is needed.

Practice

This section contains activities to reinforce the information provided in the previous section. The activities can be grouped into two main types: activities for reflection and assimilation of content and activities directed towards research, implementation of skills and strategies in multilingual settings. These activities can be undertaken individually, in pairs or small groups and / or with people from different cultural backgrounds to provide fertile grounds for discussion in class or via email. This will depend largely on the way the book is used (e.g. for self-study, as a textbook, or as support material for any course connected with intercultural communication).

Activity 1.

Read comments 1 to 5 from Boxes 4.1. to 4.5. above, and say if you agree or not, adding your own comments.

Activity 2.

Read the comments written in the section dedicated to the role of cultural differences and its effects on health care. As a Spanish citizen familiar with the healthcare system, what are the main differences you see between the American or British system as explained in the article and the Spanish system? In the case you are not Spanish, compare the comments in the article with the system in your own country.

Activity 3.

Could you define what an 'interpreter' is? Have you ever worked with (been helped by) an interpreter? How is this different from an 'ad hoc interpreter'? Do you agree with the comments in the article about ad hoc interpreters?

Activity 4.

Think about some solutions to improve intercultural communication in healthcare settings. You may think about your environment and write about some kind of cultural practice that you think social workers, doctors, judges, teachers (i.e. potential service providers) may need to know about foreign population that they are not already familiar with or that may seem strange to them.

Activity 5.

Write about some cultural practices or customs that you have observed in hospitals, courts, banks, supermarkets, schools, etc. that you think may be (or are) new or difficult to understand for people who are not familiar with this environment. Exchange your answers with other people or discuss the topic with people that you know that have contact with foreigners.

Bibliographic references and further reading

Dodd, C. (1991). *Dynamics of intercultural communication*. Dubuque, IA: Wm.C. Brown Publishers.

Ennis, S., Ríos-Vargas, M., and Albert N. (2011). "The Hispanic population: 2010". *2010 Census Briefs,* 2. Washington DC: United States Census Bureau.

Ferraro, V., Palmer K. (2005). "Differences between oral and written communication". *Speaking and arguing: the rhetoric of peace and war.* Mount Holyoke College: South Hadley, Massachusetts.

Flores G., Abreu M., Barone CP., Bachur R. and Lin H. (2012). "Errors of medical interpretation and their potential clinical consequences: a comparison of professional versus ad hoc versus no interpreters." *Annals of Emergency Medicine,* 60(5), 545-53.

Flores, G., Laws, M., Mayo, S., Zuckerman, B., Abreu M., Medina, L., and Hardt, E. (2003). "Errors in medical interpretation and their potential clinical consequences in pediatric encounters." *Pediatrics*, 111(1), 6.

Haffner, L. (2012). "Translation is not enough-interpreting in a medical setting". *The Western Journal of Medicine,* 157-257.

Hamelink, C. (1998). "Human rights: the implementation gap." *Journal of International Communication*, 5, 54-74.

Misra-Herbert, A., MD (2003). "Physician cultural competence: cross-cultural communication improves care". *Cleveland Clinic Journal of Medicine,* 70, 293- 296.

Narayanan, A. (2012). "Interpreters may help shorten hospital stays". *Chicago Tribune*. June 18th, 2012 http://articles.chicagotribune.com/2012-05-25/lifestyle/sns-rt-us-hospital-interpretersbre84o0z4-20120525_1_interpreters-patients-general-internal-medicine [Last accessed April 30th, 2014].

Olgierda F. and Heidi A. (2004). "Interpreting for the community." *Wake Forest University.* June 1st, 2012 http://lrc.wfu.edu/community_interpreting/pages/ad-hoc-interpreter.htm [Last accessed April 30th, 2014].

Secretaría General de Inmigración y Emigración. (2012). "Extranjeros residentes en España". *Ministerio de Empleo y Seguridad Social*. June 11th, 2012 http://extranjeros.empleo.gob.es/es/Estadisticas/ [Last accessed April 30th, 2014].

Sim, A. (2012). "Spain enters new recession with worse to come, says central bank". *El País: in English*. June 13th, 2012 http://elpais.com/elpais/2012/04/23/inenglish/1335192339_820649.html [Last accessed April 30th, 2014].

Tardón, L. (2009). "Los médicos españoles tienen pánico a hablar en inglés en los congresos". *El Mundo*. May 21st, 2012 http://www.elmundo.es/elmundosalud/2009/12/23/medicina/1261586856.html [Last accessed April 30th, 2014].

Traber, M. (2008). "Communication is inscribed in human nature". *World Association for Christian Communication*. June 8th, 2012.

U.S. Bureau of Labor Statistics. (2010). "Pharmacist" *U.S. Department of Labor*. May 31st, 2012.

UniversalDoctor. (2011). "Universal Doctor and Tools". June 13th, 2012 http://www.universaldoctor.com/sect/en_GB/9002/Products.html] [Last accessed April 30th, 2014].

Valero-Garcés, C. and Dergam, A. (2001). "¿Mediador social = mediador interlingüístico = Intérprete? Práctica, formación y reconocimiento del intérprete en los servicios sociales". *Sin Fronteras*, 3, 16-19.

Valero-Garcés, C. (2001d). "Estudio para determinar el tipo y calidad de la comunicación lingüística con la población extranjera en los Centros de Salud". *OFRIM, Suplementos*, 117-132.

—. (2010). "Challenging communication in doctor / non-native patient encounters. Two perspectives, three types of interaction and some proposals". *The Journal of Specialised Translation*, 14, 230.

Williams S., Weinman J. and Dale J. (1998). "Doctor-patient communication and patient satisfaction: a review". *Family Practice*, 15, 480-492.

Young, H. (2007). "Social norms" *Economics Series Working Papers*, 307, 3. University of Oxford, Department of Economics.

CHAPTER FIVE

TOPICS: INFORMED CONSENT AND THE QUALITY OF COMMUNICATION

Key Points

- Informed consent
- Legal foundations of informed consent
- Foreign population and informed consent
- Translating

Key Readings

Clark, S., Mangram, A., Ernest, D., Lebron, R. y Peralta, L. (2011). "Informed Consent: A study of the efficacy of Informed Consent and the associated role of language barriers". *Journal of Surgical Education* 68 (2): 143-147.

Galán Cortés, J.C. (1997). *El consentimiento informado del usuario de los servicios sanitarios*. Madrid: Colex.

Hunt L M and de Voogd, K. B. (2007). "Are good intentions good enough? Informed consent without trained interpreters". *J Gen Intern Med*, May 2007; 22 (5): 598-605.

Schenker Y., Wang F., Selig S. J., Ng R, Fernández A. (2007). "The impact of language barriers on documentation of informed consent at a hospital with on-site interpreter services". *Gen Intern Med*, Nov 2007; 22 Suppl 2:294-9.

5.1. Introduction. Informed Consent

This chapter deals with a specific case of communication in doctor-patient consultations: the use of Informed Consent. It is the patient's right to consent voluntarily and without coercion and with a full understanding of the procedure he/she is to undergo. Informed consent (IC), is the legal document that protects this right. However, with respect to doctor / non-native patient encounters, many questions arise, questions such as: What happens when the patient does not "understand" the text? What can the patient do when he/she does not know the language in which the consent is written? How can one exercise their right to understand and be understood? What mechanisms are in place within the Spanish health care system to enforce that right in the context of a foreign population that does not speak Spanish?

The main aim of this chapter is to analyze another dimension of the quality of communication between service providers and foreign users as investigated in previous work (Valero-Garcés 2010, 2008a,b, 2009), and to establish some conclusions that might allow us to take one step further in our study of this topic.

5.2. Informed Consent as a legal document

It is the patient's right to consent voluntarily and without coercion and with a full understanding of the procedure he / she is to undergo and the "informed consent" (IC) is therefore the legal document that protects this right. In Spain, this right is guaranteed by both national and international laws and regulations such as the Spanish Constitution, Law 14/1986 of the 25 of April on General Health, the Basic Law regulating patient autonomy and obligations pertaining to clinical information and documentation (Law 41/2002), Resolution 613/1976 and the European Council's Recommendation 779/1976.

In these and other similar documents we can find several definitions of IC.

Box 5.1.

In the Spanish Law on Health and in Article 3 of Law 41/2002 IC is defined as "the patient's free, voluntary and conscious consent expressed while of sound mind after having obtained the appropriate information so that an action affecting his health may take place."

Box 5.2.

In the eyes of the Galician Law 3/2001 Informed Consent represents "the consent expressed by the patient and demonstrated in writing after having obtained the appropriate information in order to carry out a diagnostic or therapeutic procedure that affects that individual and which involves significant, evident or considerable risks" (Guerrero Zaplana 2003: 222).

Box 5.3.

The Center of Documentation on Bioethics at the University of Navarra considers the IC to be a tool for communication between the doctor and the patient within the framework of the *lex artis*, a notion which involves "a set of medical practices which are generally accepted as appropriate to treat those who are ill at the present time", adding that "By definition the technical advances in medicine are ever changing […], just as the personal characteristics of each patient do […]".

In this sense, one might say that Informed Consent is born from the responsibility inherent to any medical procedure for which the healthcare worker may be held accountable by law (at any given time, should it become necessary). This, in turn, is directly linked to the patient's right to information and autonomy.

At first glance, these definitions of informed consent are very similar. Clearly there are points in common, but it is just as evident that some are defined in more specific terms and are therefore more restrictive in nature. This is important if we consider the significant role these texts play in legal cases involving patients and physicians. These cases allow the first party the opportunity to lodge complaints against what they consider to be negligent medical care, while the physicians can defend their position and justify the professional processes followed during the course of their work. That said, what is observed in these definitions of Informed Consent is an evolution away from the primarily paternalistic focus in the traditional doctor-patient relationship, which has generally followed along a vertical axis, towards one which is horizontal; where there is a greater degree of equality. With this shift, the physician maintains his / her obligation to offer the best care and to provide the patient with all the necessary information, but the patient is granted more individual freedom and his / her self-determination is reaffirmed when it comes time to make a decision.

5.3. The legal foundation of Informed Consent

Law 41/2002 establishes the foundations and the essential elements for the provision of Informed Consent. We will summarize this law in the following lines, referring to the work of Guerrero Zaplana (2003) for further information.

Box 5.4.

Elements for the provision of Informed consent 1. The person whose obligation it is to provide information. 2. The person who receives the information. 3. The informational content. 4. The format or the formal requirements of the IC. 5. Exceptions to the Informed Consent requirement.

The first element or party to the IC is the person whose obligation it is to provide information, a duty which falls upon the physician who is responsible for the patient or upon any professional who provides the patient with some form of medical care. According to Article 3 of the aforementioned law, the person deemed the *responsible physician* is the "professional responsible for coordinating the information and health care provided to the patient or service user and who will be the principal contact person for all matters relating to the care and information received by the patient during the provision of medical attention, without prejudice to the duties of other professionals participating in the patient's care".

The second element or party to bear in mind is the person who receives the information or, as he is referred to by Law 41/2002, the entitled party. Article 5 indicates that it is the patient who possesses the right to information. Mention is also made to "those connected to him through family ties or through domestic partnership", who also must be informed to the extent decided by the patient, either tacitly or expressly. However, there are several specific instances in which consent will not be provided by the patient. These situations arise when someone is incapable of giving his/her consent or in cases where consent is provided through a representative. There are three circumstances in which informed consent through a representative applies: 1.When the physician feels that the patient is not capable of making a decision for him/herself; 2. When the patient is legally incompetent; 3. When the patient is a minor, though there are other aspects to this that we cannot explore here (See Law 41/2002, Article 9.3.c).

The third critical element of Informed Consent is its informational content. Article 8 of Law 41/2002 specifies the interventions for which it is necessary to inform the patient and for which one must obtain his free and voluntary consent. This includes "any action pertaining to the health of the patient".

Box 5.5.

Article 4 of Spanish Law 41/2002 establishes the minimum amount of information about which the responsible physician must inform the patient, which must include "the purpose and nature of each intervention, the risks and consequences." Delving a bit deeper into this matter, the following aspects should not be overlooked:

a) Significant or important consequences resulting from the intervention.

b) Risks related to the patient's personal or professional situation.

c) Probable risks in normal circumstances, based on experience and the science of the time or those which are directly related with the type of intervention to be used.

d) Contraindications. (Law 41/2002, article 10.1)

All of these considerations seem to come together to create a rather complete and complex message for the person who must make this decision and must weigh the risks and benefits of a medical procedure. These elements provide a framework by which to evaluate the Informed Consent form, which is something we will be doing further along.

The fourth aspect of interest in our analysis is the format or the formal requirements of the IC. As a general rule, both Article 4 (in general) and Article 8.2 (in detail) of the law we have been consulting up this point, describe any information which can be presented orally. That said, exceptions to this rule are specified, which means that the written option must be used to provide information and obtain the patient's consent in cases such as "surgical intervention, invasive diagnostic and therapeutic procedures and in general, for any procedure involving risks or drawbacks resulting in a clear and foreseeable negative impact on the health of the patient" (Law 41/2002, Article 8.2). In addition, the second section of the same article specifies the need for the consent to be in writing; in the case of the procedures and the interventions detailed above and also mentions the possibility of including other types of extensions or supplementary information. Lastly, Section 4 refers to educational or research projects for which procedures done on patients can be used on the condition that there will be no ill effect the patient's health.

To conclude this section, we should mention some aspects related to the exceptions to the Informed Consent requirement.

Box 5.6.

Law 41/2002 takes into account two kinds of situations where the responsible physician need not inform the patient about the procedures he or she will undergo. These are the "classic cases of impossibility" and the "cases of therapeutic necessity", as described in Article 5 (More information in Guerrero Zaplana (2003)).

In conclusion, according to Article 10.1 of Law 41/2002, the basic elements which must always be included on this type of form are the purpose and nature of the procedure, common risks and those specific to the individual, important consequences and contraindications.

There is no general corpus of IC for the country nor is there one for the autonomous communities or even among regional hospitals or healthcare centers. Furthermore, no references exist cataloguing the quality of communication or the use of IC in cases involving patients without a good command of the official language of the country (which, in this case, is Spanish).

5.4. Contrastive analysis of the elements of Informed Consent. Study 1

Keeping in mind the elements which must be included in the IC and the lack of a general corpus, the next step will be to analyze these characteristics and the types of texts that can be found.

5.4.1. Formal characteristics of Informed Consent

Following Balaban's research (2012), three different ICs have been selected. These documents vary in terms of their content and origin, and are different, as well, for two principal reasons: Firstly, they differ in terms of their utility and frequency of use, and secondly, they come from three different hospitals, each one in a different region (or *Comunidad Autónoma*) in Spain. The ICs selected were: *Informed Consent for Egg Protein Provocation Test,* from the Pediatric Department of the Hospital Príncipe de Asturias in Alcala de Henares, Madrid, Autonomous

Community of Madrid (CAM), (referred as IC 1); *Written Consent: Local Analgesic during Labor*, from the Department of Anesthesiology and Reanimation of the University Hospital of Guadalajara (Autonomus Community of Castilla-La Mancha Regional Government (JCCM), (referred as IC 2); and *Informed Consent: Cesarean Section*, from the Autonomous Community of Valencia (referred as IC 3).

The result is the following comparative chart (Box 5.7) following the study by Balaban (2012). The table includes the characteristics from each one of the IC studied, bearing in mind the essential elements set out by the law:

Box 5.7.

<table>
<tr><th colspan="2">IC 1</th><th colspan="2">IC 2</th><th>IC 3</th></tr>
<tr><td colspan="2">1. Information about the health care facility</td><td colspan="2">1. Introduction to the health care facility</td><td>1. Identification of the authority</td></tr>
<tr><td colspan="2">2. Identification of patient/doctor and date</td><td colspan="2">2. Refusal to be informed</td><td>2. Identification and description of the process</td></tr>
<tr><td rowspan="3">3. Description of procedure</td><td>3.1. Test</td><td colspan="2" rowspan="3">3. Description of procedure (including the purpose)</td><td rowspan="3">3. Aim of the procedure and expected benefits</td></tr>
<tr><td>3.2. Aim</td></tr>
<tr><td>3.3. Result</td></tr>
<tr><td colspan="2">4. Usual risks of the procedure</td><td colspan="2">4. Consequences</td><td>4. Reasonable alternatives to this procedure</td></tr>
<tr><td colspan="2" rowspan="2">5. Personalized risks</td><td rowspan="2">5. Risks</td><td>5.1. Frequent but noncritical risks</td><td rowspan="2">5. Foreseeable consequences of doing procedure</td></tr>
<tr><td>5.2. Serious but unusual risks</td></tr>
<tr><td colspan="2">6. Possible alternatives</td><td colspan="2">6. Contraindications</td><td>6. Foreseeable consequences of not doing procedure</td></tr>
<tr><td colspan="2">7. Signatures</td><td colspan="2">7. Personalized risks</td><td>7. Frequent risks</td></tr>
<tr><td colspan="2">8. Revocation</td><td colspan="2">8. Treatments and alternative procedures</td><td>8. Infrequent risks</td></tr>
</table>

	9. Observations		9. Risks depending on patient's personal situation
	10.Statements and Signatures	10.1. Woman in labor	10. Statement of consent
		10.2. Representative	
		10.3. Responsible physician	
		10.4. Revocacion of consent	
			11. Revocation of consent

According to the structured information in Table 1, IC 1 is the least complete of the three documents, given that it is missing the last two categories of information. The other two however, are very complete and well-structured examples. IC 2 appears to be the most complete example of an informed consent form; apart from including the possibility for the patient to refuse to be informed, it also contains the greatest number of sections (taking into account subdivisions as well). Additionally, on a terminological level, it includes something noteworthy in the sense that it is the only text of the three in which the phrase *responsible physician* appears, a term established by Article 3 of the aforementioned Law on Health.

The order and subdivisions within the analyzed informed consent forms do not tend to vary by much. One section, which is without a doubt well developed in all three, is the one focusing on the risks, which are classified into different categories in each of the forms.

With respect to the formula used in the provision or revocation of the consent, IC 2 continues to be the most complete, while IC 3 stands out for its dearth of information, given that it refers only to the patient's having received and understood the doctor's explanation. However, IC 1 also includes a statement of satisfaction and specifies that along with the provision of the consent itself, opportunity has been given to ask questions or raise any doubts. IC 2 takes these elements one step further and informs the patient of the opportunity to revoke their authorization.

The situation is different, however, if we analyze the information requested from the individuals involved in the provision of the consent. In this case, IC 3 is the document that requires the most information. On the form the patient must fill in the following information: name and last name, age, address, national ID card #, and Community Health Card # (identification number corresponding to the Population Data System which is assigned to those who seek medical care in the Community of Valencia). Likewise, the doctor must indicate his / her name, last name, national ID card #, professional license # and if applicable, the identity of the legal representative and his / her relationship to the patient. The date and the signatures, both of the healthcare professional and the patient or his representative are elements which without question must also be included.

All in all, we can say without reservation that the documents selected fulfill the formal requirements. However, as we have commented previously, their variability prevents there from being any general corpus.

5.4.2. Level of language: Use of terminology

With respect to terminology, our main observation is that the level of specialization of the three texts is medium to high. Although it is certain that there are plenty of specific terms, this does not transform the document into one that would be impossible for a layperson to understand. Obviously, this observation can only be understood in a broad and universal sense, given that the limits of one's comprehension of such information are extremely relative. It will not only depend on the skill the doctor shows in explaining the procedure to the patient, but will also depend on the patient's ability to understand this information. Confronted with such a situation, the patient will be conditioned at all times by his level of study and education, work environment, social environment, health and emotional status or previous experience and even more so if the consent is given in a language other than his native tongue or if he must rely on the abilities of the interpreter who, in an ideal or hypothetical situation, would be there to mediate an encounter of this kind.

Other factors that can influence one's comprehension of medical terminology are the level of specialty associated with the procedure or treatment to be performed and the patient's level of education. To this we should add another factor which has already been mentioned, which is the command of the language in the case of foreign patients, as well as other factors which we will examine further along.

To use an example of two fairly common surgical interventions, there will always be those who know that it means to remove the appendix or the tonsils, but who are not aware that in specialized terms these procedures are respectively referred to as "appendectomy" and "tonsillectomy". Likewise, in cases of very rare diseases or interventions generally unknown to the public, there will be patients who have never heard of the term or treatment for their condition until the doctor informs them of the diagnosis. In any case, the knowledge about medicine (or anatomy, at least) that the general population is assumed to possess as a result of their education is never particularly consistent. This knowledge depends on each person and their level of education, as well as where they received this education. This is even truer in the case of people of foreign origin or those who have been educated in a different country or educational system.

5.4.3. Form and content

The three ICs share certain common characteristics in how they are written, both in terms of their linguistic and extra-linguistic elements. However, when considering the task of translating these documents into another language, a more detailed analysis reveals a series of difficulties to bear in mind.

1. Spelling and typographical errors in the original text (OT). Since this is a text with a clear practical objective – to inform the patient and to aid the responsible physician in providing non-routine explanations – these errors tend to go unnoticed in the original text and only cause a real problem in certain cases when they create ambiguity and affect the comprehension of the message. For example, in IC 1 we find *moderared* instead of *moderated* or *alternatibe* instead of *alternative* and in IC 3 the Latin expression is written as *quod functionem* instead of *quod funcionem*. Likewise, as we see in the following excerpt of text, this last consent also contains an error in spelling, resulting in a lack of agreement in number: "Be aware that the risks (*riesgos*) are more frequent (*frecuente*) the lesser their severity […]"; the adjective *frecuente* (frequent) should be plural since it refers to the noun *riesgos (risks).*

Other errors are related to punctuation. This is the case in the following example in which we find a phrase beginning with a subordinate conjunction *que (that)* directly after another phrase ending in a period:

> *I STATE that I have been adequately informed by the physician and have been given as much notice as possible regarding the procedure to be performed, as well as about the risks, complications, anticipated benefits and alternatives. *That* I know and assume the risks and consequences that could result from or be caused by the aforementioned procedure, during labor or due to complications from the intervention.

In this case, it would have been best to use a semicolon to correctly separate the two phrases. Likewise, IC 3 also contains several sentences that create problems due to the improper use of comas (due to excessive use or lack thereof), which can be observed in the following example where a qualifying adjective is separated from its noun, even getting in the way of the predicate and the direct object. "On occasions the delivery of the fetus is aided by the use of a vacuum extractor which leaves the corresponding, temporary mark."

2. Grammatical errors appear in the original text. In this category we find incorrect usage related to agreement. Errors in subject / verb agreement or gender agreement seem to be the most prevalent and give way to ambiguity or even cause the text to be incomprehensible. In point 7 of IC 3 we see an example: Ambiguity is generated when discussing one type of risk of a cesarean. As a result, a greater effort must be made to comprehend the message and, in the case of the translator/interpreter, to convert it into the target language. The content of the statement is the following: "On some occasions they can (pueden) produce more serious effects such as a blood clotting disorder (DIC) or generalized infection." At first glance there doesn't appear to be a problem, but the key here resides in the fact that there is no explicit subject and that the section is entitled "Uncommon Risks", which gives way to two different interpretations. Although both the phrase and the verb "pueden" (can) are plural, the phrase does not make very much sense from a semantic point of view. Thus, a subject should have been included, the verb should have been made singular, or the phrase could have been formulated using the passive reflexive with the word *effects* as a reference. The latter would have given way to "On some occasions more serious effects can be produced…", which would have been grammatically correct.

Also in point 4 of the same IC we encounter a problem due to grammatical incoherence stemming from the corruption of the prepositional regimen. Due to the influence of the preceding parenthesis, the preposition *de* (of) is added to a phrase that is part of a complex subject: "[Carrying out the procedure] is not without reasonable risks given that it involves a combined labor/delivery (since this procedure involves a certain type of this) and *of* a surgical intervention." Simply removing the preposition *of* takes care of the problem.

The lack of coherence is apparent on other occasions as well, especially when the documents alternate the use of the word *patient* in the masculine (*el paciente*) with that of the feminine (*la paciente*). Additionally, if we consider the fact that, at least in the case of IC 2 and 3, the patient must always be female, it is more understandable and even advisable that this commonly used noun appear in its feminine form and that this be maintained throughout the entire text to avoid further complication.

IC 1 also contains an error of this type in the portion where reference is made to the egg protein provocation test. Literally, the text and the translation reads:

Box 5.8.

OT: "El resultado de esta prueba puede ser negativo: con una ausencia de síntomas negativos y por lo tanto el niño será considerado tolerante a la comida, o positiva: exhibiendo síntomas adversos inmediatos". (The underlined is mine)

TT: "*The result* (*el resultado)* of this test can be NEGATIVE (*negativo):* with an absence of adverse symptoms and, therefore, the child will be considered tolerant to the food, or POSITIVE (*positiva):* exhibiting immediate adverse symptoms".

The most logical explanation for this incoherence is that the adjective *positiva* (fem.) ('positive') has been associated with the noun *prueba* (fem) ('test')*;* however, after choosing to have *negative* (masc.) agree *resultado (masc* ('result'), such wording proves incorrect and the adjective must take the masculine form.

This ambiguity or lack of clarity is also evident in the example of IC 2 and the 'patient's signature' *(firma del paciente).* The gender of the noun patient *(paciente*) is not specified although it is known that in this case the person who signs the consent as the patient can only be a woman, regardless of whether the legal representative is a man or woman. As a result, the translator is forced to choose between one form and the other; for example, in the case of Romanian, opting for the feminine form of the equivalent: "semnătura pacientei" (patient's signature).

3. Cultural elements interfering with meanings. This is the case with the reference to *tortilla* (IC 1). Although the text does not specify if it is the typically Spanish *tortilla de patata* ("potato omelet") that is being referred to or if it is another type of omelet, such as one containing only eggs, anyone in Spain automatically interprets this term as the former. One possibility is to make an adaptation or to seek the cultural equivalent in the target language. In Romanian for example, as Balaban comments, the more general equivalent *omletă* ('omelet') might be used.

4. Formatting. Another challenge facing the translator is how to handle images, drawings, graphs and previously established formats. One example from Informed Consents analyzed is the handling of logos. In order to be included in the target language in the final text, the logos of Hospital Príncipe de Asturias, CAM and Salud Madrid must be manipulated in an image editor in order to directly edit any words in the original language.

5. Handling of content. It is interesting to note as well that, apart from the differences in geographic area, these ICs are different in other ways which illustrates the variability we have been referring to. In this manner IC 3, although it comes from a medical department similar to that of IC 2, takes a very different approach and is characterized by the superficiality of the statements comprising the portion where the actual consent is provided.

In terms of positive elements and general content, IC 1 and 2 come from Autonomous Communities which are close to one another and which continue to share common ties in some areas. Our research is focused precisely on these communities and although these IC belong to different medical specialties, they have many characteristics in common, which is to the advantage of the translator who frequently works with this type of document. Hence, for example, in the portion of the consent where the patient makes his statements and gives his authorization, we find a standard phrase used in informed consent: "I am satisfied with the information received, I have been able to ask all the questions I considered appropriate and all doubts raised have been clarified to me." The only aspects of the phrase that vary are that in IC 2, because the subject is in the feminine form, the adjective satisfied appears as *satisfecha* and with respect to the propositional regimen of this adjective; the preposition *con* is changed to *de.* This type of repetition is of great advantage to the translator or even to the interpreter that frequently handles texts of this type because it gives him / her added confidence and it saves time and effort when carrying out his/her work.

5.4.4. Translating Informed Consent

Elements in the original text that might cause problems to the translator:

1. The lack of quality in the original text shows that a more diligent editing of the texts used in healthcare is necessary in order to avoid the number of errors we have demonstrated here. These errors

usually create extra work down the road for the translator. They can also cause confusion for the interpreter who must perform a sight translation of the document, which means additional time will be required in order to decipher the message and a higher level of concentration will be necessary so as to avoid making mistakes while transmitting the message into the target language.

2. Lack of consideration for the person receiving the information. Textually, the IC should not pose any kind of great difficulty in terms of style and register, unless there are errors in the original text that might make it more difficult to understand and that could complicate the subsequent transfer of the text from one language to another. Present experience indicates that once one is familiar with the mechanics of this type of text, translation ceases to be a difficult task. In its essence this type of document will always be the same, which compensates for the more than likely terminological obstacles that are inherent to every medical specialty. Alternatively, given the practical nature of these texts, it is necessary to always keep the reader of the text in mind and to try to transmit the message as clearly and transparently as possible. This is indicated by the results of Balaban's study and the preliminary conclusions drawn from other studies still in progress in the Chinese-Spanish and Arabic-Spanish language pairs within the Master's Program in Intercultural Communication offered by the University of Alcala, as well as by the recommendations of the healthcare workers themselves.
3. Imbalances exist in the availability and use of resources for translators. This partly depends on the language combination involved and the translator's own abilities with respect to documentation, searches and the use of translation tools. Something that was also brought to light was the utility of having access to specialized texts in any format in order to create databases that might be helpful to translators. Nor should we forget that another important source of information can be found in the healthcare specialists themselves.
4. The interdisciplinary nature of translation. The transfer of a text from one language to another demands that the translator be in contact with a multitude of areas which, at first glance, may seem to have little to do with one another. However, if one wishes to translate well, he/she must be closely connected with all these different areas. Translation does not only involve providing a service to the service provider or user, but also requires one to have

exposure to the related fields of knowledge (such as, in this case, medicine, law, cultural studies, foreign languages, TIC, layout and design, etc.) that help the translator to carry out his work with the highest level of quality and professionalism.

5.5. Multilingual populations and the use of Informed Consent

As a way to illustrate the difficulties that foreign populations might face during the Informed Consent process, two research projects were conducted. The starting hypotheses were the following:

1. The concept of Informed Consent is fairly unknown to both the native Spaniard and those of foreign origin. Special focus was given to the Romanian population, since that is the largest foreign population in the area where the study was conducted;
2. As a text, the IC presents serious difficulties for those who do not dominate the language in which it is written and this prevents the text from being properly understood.

Of the two different studies, one survey was conducted to determine what knowledge people in the area had of the IC. Alternatively, another survey was conducted among the foreign population in order to find out what difficulties they had in understanding the IC. A brief summary of these studies follows.

5.5.1 Study 1. Empirical study on the use of the IC by the NSSP

In her study, Balaban (2012) designed a survey in Spanish that was then translated into Romanian and was distributed both over the Internet and in person in several cities and towns in the Community of Madrid (CM) and Guadalajara (JCCM). The survey contained questions related to the informed consent form and process, how many had read or signed one in their own name or as representative of a family member, in which country they had to do so, what intervention or treatment was involved, how the doctor behaved, if they felt there was any difference between a translator and an interpreter and if so, if they could explain what that difference was.

In the part aimed at Spaniards, they were also asked to choose one of the options provided related to having to undergo a procedure in a country where they did not know the language (this question also appeared in the portion aimed at the rest of the population) and were asked if they had ever been cared for by a healthcare provider who did not share their language and if so, if there had been problems in the communication. At the end they were given the chance to add any personal comments.

Likewise, those of foreign origin were asked if anyone had ever offered these options to facilitate communication when undergoing a procedure in Spain, who this person had been (several available options), how they would feel having the help of a professional translator or interpreter in the hypothetical situation of an intervention or hospitalization and if they would like to add any comments.

Table 5.3 gathers statistics in terms of the scope of the survey and subject participation, which just surpasses two thirds of all distributed questionnaires. This is a fairly positive value keeping in mind that the study was conducted in a relatively short time span.

Box 5.9.

Format	Number of questionnaires distributed	Number of responses to questionnaires	Participation rate
Electronic	100	77	76.2%
Paper	50	24	48%
Total	150	101	67.3%

Table 5.3: Data on people surveyed and their responses.

Personal variables included in the survey were sex, nationality, length of time in Spain (in the case of the foreign citizens) and age, which consisted of four age ranges: under twenty years old, between twenty and thirty five, between thirty five and fifty, and over fifty years old. In any case, it is important to emphasize that both in the online and written versions of the survey, these questions were optional.

With respect to nationalities, the percentages, which were calculated based on the 101 participants who answered this question, show that the majority of those sampled were Spanish, with a percentage of about 61.4% (62 people), followed by almost 30.7% or 31 of those surveyed of Romanian origin. For other nationalities, three participants were French, two were Belgian, one was Saudi Arabian, one was Polish and one was Thai. In addition, a calculation was made in order to determine the approximate length of time that the foreign citizens surveyed had been in Spain. In order to simplify the process, any period of time of 6 months or more was rounded up to a year, while anything below 6 months was rounded down. The result obtained shows that the 39 foreigners surveyed had resided in Spain for a period of 7.3 years on average, with the longest time being 22 years and the shortest, 5 months.

As for the results of interest to us here, regarding the question of whether or not they knew what IC was, the results in Graph 1 reveal a rather high level of knowledge. However, there is quite a margin of difference in the results between the Spaniards and the Romanians.

The negative responses account for a very low rate, which is a very hopeful indicator of the knowledge people have about tools such as Informed Consent, meant to safeguard and protect their health.

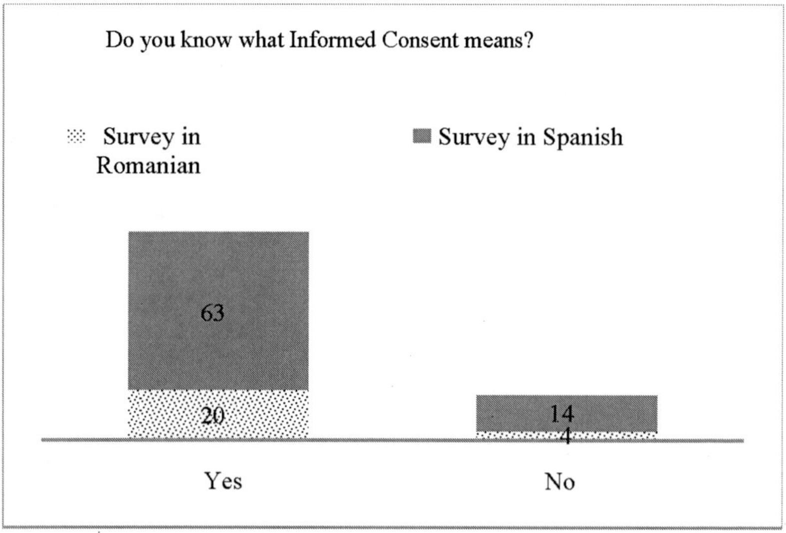

Graph 5.1: What is Informed Consent?

The next question of interest was if the subject had ever signed an IC form (Graph 5.2). Our data indicates that the majority had not done so.

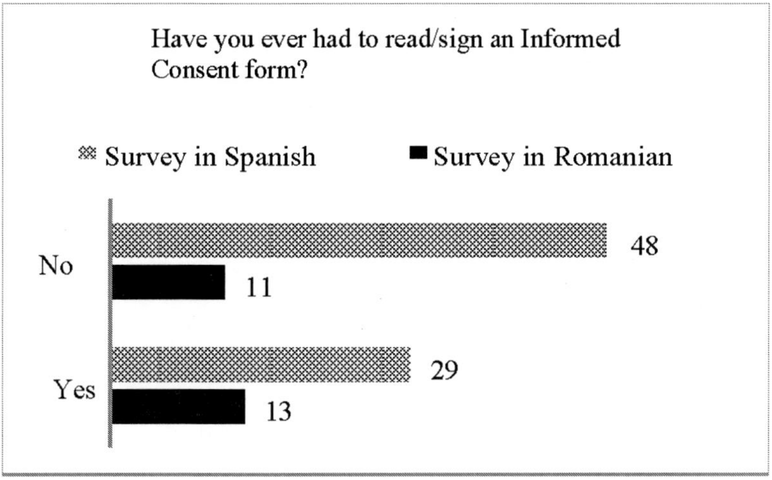

Graph 5.2: Read/sign an Informed Consent form

If we continue investigating into those who responded affirmatively to this question, when asked where the signing took place, the majority indicated that in Spain (On the questionnaire in Spanish, 27 in Spain and 2 in another country and on the questionnaire in Romanian, 15 in Spain and 5 in Romania).

Regarding the reason for having read and signed the consent, the results are the following:

- Survey in Spanish: surgical intervention (seven times), (surgical) extraction of wisdom teeth (five times), allergy test (2 times), vaccine administration (two times), upper GI endoscopy (two times), meniscus surgery, appendectomy, lithotripsy operation, administration of oral contrast agent for an MRI, anesthesia (both local and general, 5 examples total), gamma camera cardiac imaging, medication with certain risks and invasive medical testing, ultrasound, radioactive iodine, diagnostic procedures, MRI arthrography of the ankle, gallbladder removal, epidural for labor/cesarean section.
- Survey in Romanian: tympanoplasty, cholecystectomy, hysterosalpingography, endoscopy, routine blood tests, surgical intervention (without further specification), general medicine (idem).

This information supports Sanchez's comments (2012) that the three specialty areas where Informed Consent is most needed are: surgery, anesthesia and oncology. The first two areas are the most frequent in the above lists. It should also be pointed out that a great number of the procedures listed above involve diagnostic skills. That, in spite of the fact that the population sample is not large in number, the responses reflect significant variety, which would be worthy of analysis in future studies.

When asked how the doctor conducted himself or herself before the consent form had been signed (in the case of those who had done so), the following values were obtained from each of the five alternatives given (the first number corresponds to the survey in Spanish while the second reflects the data obtained from the questionnaire in Romanian):

- "All the content on the form was explained to me in detail": 8 in Spanish versus 5 in Romanian;
- "I was explained the contents of the form summarily": 15 in Spanish versus 5 in Romanian;
- "Nothing on the form was explained to me": 2 in Spanish versus 1 in Romanian;
- "I wasn't even shown the form, I was only asked for my signature": 0 in Spanish versus 1 in Romanian;
- "Other (Please specify)": 53 in Spanish versus 12 in Romanian.

Although the number obtained from this last option represents the majority in both cases, the lack of specificity and the fact that the numbers correspond closely to Graph 3 lead us to conclude that those who had never read or signed an IC form checked this option anyway (so as not to leave the question blank.) One person even used the extra space at the bottom to clarify that he had chosen both the first and the second option. Since the question was multiple choice, he would not have been able to choose both options had he not had the possibility to include his comment below. However, the additional comments from the few individuals surveyed who did provide more detailed commentary deserve consideration, and it is for this reason we have included further quotes below:

- "I don't remember but I think I was given a paper with further explanation, explanation that was more clear. [sic] but it wasn't Informed Consent."
- "I was asked to read it at home and to bring it back signed."
- "We were not shown the form but the procedure and its risks were explained to us and afterwards my signature was requested."
- "The first option and since I still didn't understand, he made a drawing".

Another key question for our study had to do with whether the foreign participants that had undergone an intervention in Spain requiring an IC to be signed had received someone's help with the communication. In this case, only 8 of the 15 foreigners answered the question, with 7 negative responses for 1 positive response. When asked to specify who the person was by choosing from the different options provided, those surveyed marked "a family member: father/mother" and "a friend/acquaintance." This data contrasts with previous studies which had indicated (Valero-Garcés 2008 a, 2008b, 2010) that migrants usually are accompanied by different people who are linked to them in some way and who perform the interpreting.

In this study, the number of people with someone to help them communicate is three times less than the number of people who had no such person available to perform said task. This number can be explained in two ways: the individual surveyed did not need anyone thanks to the fact that he/she knew Spanish or did need someone, but it was not possible for anyone to accompany him, whether that person be a member of his family or circle of friends, an acquaintance or community member, or professional translator/interpreter whose services were not included among those offered by the patient's medical facility.

Depending on the perspective from which one views the situation, this might be cause for celebration; it could mean that foreigners are more integrated and can clearly and independently communicate with healthcare professionals. However, on the contrary, it might be cause for alarm in the case of foreign individuals who do not speak Spanish (or who don't have sufficient command of the language) don't have anyone to help them. Of course, it also suggests that there is a lack of translators and interpreters, be they members of the hospital or heathcare clinic staff or intermittent translators/interpreters (whose services are used according to demand).

Finally, in terms of personal preferences for the provisions of Informed Consent, according to the responses shown in Graph 5.3, the most heavily-weighted preference among those surveyed would be to receive the IC form in their own language and to also have translation and interpreting services available.

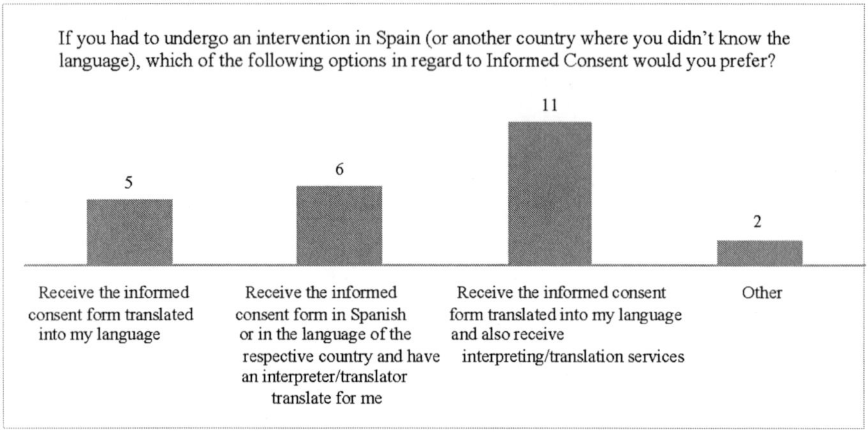

Graph 5.3: Options for Informed Consent forms

5.5.2. Study 2. Understanding translated Informed Consent among migrants

The second study was conducted by Taibi (2006). I agree with Taibi (2006: 187) that public service translation/interpreting is functional translation/interpreting and therefore, its functionality must be an important criteria, both in order to guarantee effective communication and as a means to evaluate if translation/interpreting is fulfilling its role. Stated another way, from our study, if a patient who does not speak Spanish must sign an informed consent form in order to undergo a surgical intervention but cannot understand either the original version or its translation, one would expect not only the act of communication to fail, but also to halt the medical/institutional procedure.

In his research Taibi (2006) presents data on the difficulties people had understanding the IC that was translated from Spanish into Arabic and English and distributed to migrant speakers according to the language they use in Spain (Moroccans in Arabic, Sub-Saharans (Nigerians, Ghanaians and Liberians) in English and Spaniards in Spanish). The chosen method was a survey in which the respondents had to read an informed consent form (in Spanish, Arabic or English, according to their place of origin) and underline any word that they could not understand.

Informed Consent (*IC for thoracotomy-thoracoscopy*) was chosen at random from a corpus of informed consents translated by the FITISpos research group from the University of Alcalá. The survey was conducted in an area of the Henares Corridor (Madrid and Guadalajara). A total of 210 participants took part (70 Arabs, 70 Sub-Saharans and 70 Spaniards); completely at random (in the case of the last group, at random but also based on certain conditions in the case of the first groups, Arabs and Sub-Saharans), who were asked if they had been born in Spain or in their country of ethnic origin, if they had spoken Spanish before coming to Spain, and if Arabic or English was their preferred language or *lingua franca* after arriving in Spain. In the same survey, the respondents filled out information regarding sex, age, nationality, and level of education. This last variable was believed to be important due to how it may affect comprehension of the IC form, just as the conclusions indicate:

With respect to nationality, the Arab participants were all from Morocco while the group of English speaking participants was divided among Nigerians (46), Ghanaians (13) and Liberians (11).

The main results related to the topic of our investigation indicated the following:

1. Some participants turned out to be illiterate. This meant that the utility of a translation in these cases (30%, 21.42% and 0% respectively) is null, unless another person were called upon to read the form to the patient or to do a sight translation.
2. The maximum number of underlined words (that were incomprehensible) varies significantly among those who supposedly were speakers of Spanish (6), English (19) and Arabic (24), not counting those who were illiterate.
3. While the words that were underlined in Spanish are part of medical terminology (thoracotomy, thoracoscopy, braquial plexus, pneumothorax, empiema, and dehiscence), in the case of English and Arabic, apart from medical terminology, two more word groups were included: on one hand, words used in the medical context, but which have become commonplace (eg. esophagus, diaphragm, incision, blood vessels, hemorrhage, etc.) and on the other hand, words from non-specialized language (undergo, hole, introduction, supervisors, after, etc.).

In conclusion, the results from this study confirm our hypothesis that the translated institutional texts (in this case, the IC) would not be effective forms of communication in many cases, due to the sociocultural reality of the patients and above all, the linguistic reality within their communities.

Alternatively, it demonstrates that since the target language is not the native language of these patients, their degree of linguistic and communicative competency in these languages varies from case to case and is also influenced by their level of education. In the case of Spanish, as the study by Valero and Taibi (2005) points out, much of the medical terminology has become commonplace thanks to education and easier access to information. However, in migrant communities medical terminology generally remains accessible only to an elite group of people that does not even include all professionals (many of them only have a command of medical terms in English or French).

All in all, the primary results related with the topic of this investigation indicate that, in order of importance, the greatest difficulties related to terminology – not including those who are illiterate – are the following:

- Comprehension of specialized medical expressions and terms (eg. "Thoracotomy").
- Comprehension of commonplace words used in the medical context (e.g. "Esophagus", "hemorrhage").
- Comprehension of non-specialized terms (e.g. "holes", "supervisors")
- Degree of linguistic and communicative competence in these languages when they are not the speaker's native language.

5.6. Conclusions and suggestions

Now that we have performed an in-depth examination of Informed Consent, covering a wide range of essential elements for the study of this legal-medical tool in its entirety, the time has come to present the conclusions that have emerged and try to offer some solutions and suggestions for the future.

The IC form is a legal tool for both doctor and patient which is guaranteed by several national and international laws. A comparative study of the ICs from different autonomous communities and from different medical departments reveals that the documents meet the basic rules and conditions and that they all share the same general characteristics but that there also exists a great diversity which prevents the existence of a national corpus.

Having analyzed the ICs, the goal of the second part of the paper was dedicated to the study of how IC relates to migrant populations and to attempt to understand its use and degree of effectiveness. There were several tasks that were undertaken: A series of IC were analyzed and translated and a survey was conducted – in Spanish and also in Romanian, given that this is the largest foreign group in the area where the study was conducted – on the use of the IC with the aim of contrasting the data. Alternatively, a study was also conducted on the effectiveness of the translated IC.

The first task revealed that despite the uniformity of the IC in terms of structure and content, it poses some problems for the translator due to typographical, grammatical and punctuation errors and raises a series of terminological and cultural challenges that can create problems during translation.

Despite the small group sampled for the second task- the creation, distribution and analysis of the survey – several conclusions can be drawn from the responses gathered:

- the concept of Informed Consent is fairly well-known;
- the length of many of the free answers indicates that there is interest in this topic;
- the use of Informed Consent is frequent in the medical field described by the subjects;
- individuals of foreign origin do not attend medical appointments accompanied by someone else from their environment as was originally assumed. This could be due to difficulty in making this happen (lack of time, long distances, scheduling incompatibility, etc.) or could mean that their command of Spanish allows them to go by themselves.

The third task performed reveals that there are other factors which affect the translated texts and that these texts do not always communicate as well as one assumes. Rather, a better adaptation of the medical language is called for in order to meet the needs and comprehension level of the patients, even when there is only one language involved.

To conclude and in light of these results, some recommendations should be made:

Box 5.10.

1. Create a corpus of consents and individual resources (glossaries, templates, data bases, etc.) using these types of texts.
2. Include explanation of textual typology/category in the educational guides for specialized classes both in health sciences and translation and interpreting studies.
3. Enable communication between the foreign population and the health care providers (and the proper use of the IC) by devising a plan to create some mechanisms for the proper implementation of Informed Consent process and, to the extent that it is possible, create a multidisciplinary committee to oversee this topic and everything related to it.
4. Facilitate the creation of other mechanisms based on existing needs such as the hiring of professional translators and interpreters or the use of telephone interpreting in healthcare centers.
5. Facilitate the education of both health care workers and medical service users regarding their right to give and receive adequate and sufficient information so as to ensure their autonomy in the decisions affecting their health and to inform them about the role of Informed Consent within the framework of the health care available to them.
6. Insist that the administration take the initiative to establish measures to facilitate communication with the foreign population. This will not only help the patients so that they might enjoy better access and exceptional care, but will be of advantage to the administration as well.

Proof of the last statement is the study conducted by Clark et al (2011), which shows that interpreting services end up being less costly to hospitals and mean lower bills for patients since these services help to avoid repeated or prolonged hospitalizations resulting from communication problems with the foreign patient.

All in all, Informed Consent is at certain times a key component in the communication between doctor and patient and is the patient's right, forming part of the whole set of actions comprising healthcare. Once we understand the benefits of the work of translation and interpreting professionals, particularly in the healthcare arena and in the public services in general, we will be closer to taking a great step forward for society as a whole.

Practice

This section contains activities to reinforce the information provided in the previous section. The activities can be grouped into two main types: activities for reflection and assimilation of content and activities directed towards research, implementation of skills and strategies in multilingual settings. These activities can be undertaken individually, in pairs or small groups and / or with people from different cultural backgrounds to provide fertile grounds for discussion in class or via email. This will depend largely on the way the book is used (e.g. for self-study, as a textbook, or as support material for any course connected with intercultural communication).

Activity 1.

As explained in the article, Informed Consents are legal documents. Balaban's research shows that one of the main difficulties patients have with IC are related to the use of specialized vocabulary. Look for at least ten words related to the medical setting and make a four column list using the specialized term and the colloquial word in both English and Spanish. For example: Anginas- tonsils

Activity 2.

First, read an IC in English and another one in Spanish and copy at least 10 words related to the legal setting or formal language that you may think a person with a basic knowledge of Spanish and / or basic formal education might have problem with. Secondly, look for synonyms of the words chosen.
Lastly, provide a translation for both English and Spanish words.

Activity 3.

Compare an Informed Consent in English with one in Spanish or any other language you know. Write a comment about the differences and similarities.

Activity 4.

Translate the Informed Consent into another language.

Bibliographic references and further reading

Balaban, C. (2012). *Investigación sobre consentimientos informados. Comparación de la situación entre España y Rumania*. [Unpublished Master's Thesis]. Universidad de Alcalá, Madrid, Spain.

Benavides, F.G., Nolasco, A., Jiménez, L., Gonzáles, C., López, J.M., Pérez, E. et al. (1987). "Aplicación y Validez de un Cuestionario para Medir la Satisfacción de los Usuarios de un Centro de Salud". *Aten Primaria*, 4(2), 91-95.

Byrne, J., Napier, A. and Cuschieri, A. (1988). "How informed is signed consent?" *BMJ,* 296, 839-840.

Clark, S., Mangram, A., Ernest, D., Lebron, R. and Peralta, L. (2011). "Informed Consent: A study of the efficacy of Informed Consent and the associated role of language barriers". *Journal of Surgical Education,* 68(2), 143-147.

Finkelstein, D., Smith, M.K., Faden, R. (1993). "Informed consent and medical ethics". *Arch. Opthalmology,* 111(3), 324-326.

Galán Cortés, J.C. (1997). *El Consentimiento Informado del Usuario de los Servicios Sanitarios*. Madrid: Colex.

García Valverde, M.D., Girela Molina, B. (2011). "Consentimiento informado: efectividad del mismo en la asistencia sanitaria a extranjeros". *Revista de Treball, Economía i Societat*, 60. Castellón: Comité Econòmic i Social de la Comunitat Valenciana.

Guerrero Zaplana, J. (2003). *Las Reclamaciones por la Defectuosa Asistencia Sanitaria: Doctrina, Jurisprudencia, Legislación y Formularios*. Valladolid: Lex Nova.

Gyomber, D., Lawrentschuk, N., Wong, P., Parker, F. and Bolton, D.M. (2010). "Improving informed consent for patients undergoing radical prostatectomy using multimedia techniques: a prospective randomized crossover study". *BJU International.*

Herrero de Dios, A.; Reyes Martín, A.; García Areces, F. (2000). "Consentimiento Informado en un Área de Atención Primaria". *Atención Primaria*, 25(9) 61-9.

Hunt, L.M. and De Voogd, K. B. (2007). "Are good intentions good enough? Informed consent without trained interpreters". *J Gen Intern Med*, 22(5), 598-605.

Jansà, J.M. (2008). "Políticas de salud pública e inmigración". In García Roca, J. and Lacomba, J. (Eds.) *Inmigración en la Sociedad Española: Una Radiografía Multidisciplinar.* Barcelona: Editorial Bellaterra, 865-874.

Krosin, M.T., Klitzman, R., Levin, B., Cheng, J. and Ranney, M.L. (2006). "Problems in comprehension of informed consent in rural and peri-urban Mali, West Africa". *Clinical Trials*.

Llosada Gistau, J., Vallverdú Duch, I., Miró Orpinell, M., Pijem Serra, C. and Guarga Rojas, A. (2012). "Acceso y uso de los servicios sanitarios por parte de los pacientes inmigrantes: la voz de los profesionales". *Atención Primaria* 44(2), 82-88.

Marshall, P.A., Adebamowo, C.A., Adeyemo, A.A., Ogundiran, T.O., Vekich, M., Strenski, T., Zhou, J., Prewitt, T.E., Cooper, R.S., Rotimi, C.N. (2006). "Voluntary participation and informed consent to international genetic research". *American Journal of Public Health*.

Meisel, A., Roth, L. (1981) "What we do and do not know about informed consent?" *Jama*, 246(21), 2473-2477.

Olver, I.N., Whitford, H.S., Denson, L.A., Peterson M,J. and Olver, S.I. (2009). "Improving informed consent to chemotherapy: a randomized controlled trial of written information versus an interactive multimedia". *Patient Education and Counselling.*

Pajares, M. (2007). *Inmigrantes del Este: Procesos Migratorios de los Rumanos*. Barcelona: Icaria.

Salinas de Frías, C. (2008). "Problemas de salud de la población inmigrante y su relación con el sistema sanitario". In Salinas de Frías, A. (Ed.) *Inmigración e integración: aspectos sociales y legales*. Madrid: Ediciones Sequitur, 55-76.

Schenker, Y., Wang, F., Selig, S.J., Ng, R. and Fernández, A. (2007). "The impact of language barriers on documentation of informed consent at a hospital with on-site interpreter services". *Gen Intern Med*, 22(Suppl 2), 294-9.

Simón Lorda, P. and Concheiro, L. (1993). "El Consentimiento Informado: Teoría y Práctica II". *Med Clin (Barc)*, 101(5), 174-182.

___ (1993). "El Consentimiento Informado: Teoría y Práctica I". *Med Clin (Barc)*, 100(17), 659-663.

___(1995). "El Consentimiento Informado y la Enfermería: Modelo Integral". *Jano*, 55-65.

Taibi, M. (2006). "Estudio de la utilidad de traducciones para los servicios públicos." In García Blanco, P. and Martino, P. (Eds.) *Traducción y Multiculturalidad.* Universidad Complutense: Servicio de Publicaciones, 187-193.

Tatum Krank, J., Shaykevich, Sh., Lipsitz, and S. and Soleymani, L. (2011). "Patient predictors of colposcopy comprehension of Consent among English- and Spanish-speaking Women". *Women's Health Issues*, 21(1), 80–85.

Vaccarino, J. (1978). "Consent, informed consent and the consent form". *New England Journal of Medicine*, 298(8), 455.

CHAPTER SIX

NEGOTIATION OF MEANING IN MEDICAL CONSULTATIONS

Key Points

- Institutional Discourse
- Medical Consultation Structure
- Doctors'-Patients' Interaction Mechanism
- Functions of *small talk* (STK) in Medical Consultations

Key Readings

Atkinson, P. (1999). "Medical discourse, evidentiality and the construction of professional responsibility". S. Sarangi and C. Roberts (eds.), *Talk, Work, and Institutional Order: Discourse in Medical, Mediation and Management Settings*, New York, Mouton de Gruyter, 75-106.

Long, A. (1983). "Linguistic and conversational adjustments to non-native speakers". *Studies in Second Language Acquisition* 5 (2), 177-193.

Maynard, D. W. (1991). "On the interactional and institutional bases of asymmetry in clinical discourse". *American Journal of Sociology* 92, 448-95.

Mishler, E. G. (1994). "The struggle between the voice of medicine and the voice of the lifeworld". P. Conrad y R. Kern (eds.), *The Sociology of Health and Illness: Critical Perspectives*, New York, St. Martin's, 288-300.

Thompson, T. L. (1994). "Interpersonal communication and health care". M. Knapp y G. R. Miller (eds.), *Handbook of Interpersonal Communication*, Thousands Oaks, CA, Sage, 696-725.

6.1. Introduction*

This chapter will focus on providing an analysis of the medical consultation and how meaning is negotiated in this institutional context using a very specific, but extremely relevant type of discourse known as *small talk*.

The studies on *small talk* (STK) in institutional settings reveal that, just as in other more familiar settings, STK performs different functions and is part of what forms the delicate tapestry that is conversation. Many institutional and professional undertakings are built upon or conducted using language (oral or written) as a means of communication. At the same time, these modes of expression help to identify the protagonists and reveal their discursive competence, which they employ in order to meet their objectives.

6.2. Medical consultation

The medical consultation adheres to a protocol and has a systematicity that, following upon the work of Heritage (1997) and Drew and Sorjonen (1997), can be summarized in three points: (a) The participants have specific roles, (b) There are a series of limitations which are specific to the institutional context, and (c) There are inferential frameworks and specific procedures associated with each institution.

In turn, the general structure of the doctor-patient interaction during the medical consultation includes the following sections (See Borrell, 2004):

Box 6.1.

Medical consultation structure
Initial Greetings
Assessment and discussion of how the patient is doing
Discussion and prescription of treatment and/or technical testing
Goodbyes

To the above sections, we should add two more points, as they are interwoven throughout the general structure of the consultation. These are casual interjections or *small talk* (STK) and the discussions which are related to official procedures or to institutional functions rather than to the original reason for the visit. In the following pages, the goal will be to attempt to answer two main questions: (a) In what sections and according to which functions does STK occur? and (b) Does the modification of the general structure or the speakers' participation also imply changes in the role and distribution of STK during the medical consultation?

The changes the Spanish society and healthcare system have undergone due to the arrival of foreigners who speak other languages and come from other cultures have also produced a modification of the standard structure of this type of institutional interaction, thus breaking the routine that facilitates consultations and keeps within the constraints of meeting time and space as determined by the Spanish healthcare system.

The corpus of conversations used for this study mainly come from recordings taken from several health care centers in the Corredor del Henares (an area located between northern Madrid and Guadalajara) during the years 2004-2006. For this study, we have analyzed a total of 20 conversations divided into two groups: 1. Medical consultation – Spanish patient; 2. Medical consultation – Foreign patient with good command of Spanish (1). At times we have also used fragments of conversations from the work of Díaz Martínez (2002).

With respect to the method followed, it is a qualitative study based on the structure of the medical consultation in which examples of STK taken from the corpus of conversations are analyzed in order to illustrate the different functions of STK in this specific context. Two types of consultations are analyzed and contrasted: Spanish doctor – Spanish patient and Spanish doctor – Foreign patient.

6.3. Small talk in the medical consultation

Small talk (STK) or phatic talk has been approached from many different disciplines (sociolinguistic, semantic, pragmatic, discourse analysis, communication studies). However, up until recently it was considered to be a form of conventional and peripheral speech or, in other words, to have no value of its own. The papers from the compilation by Coupland (2000), among others, have helped to eliminate such ideas and to assign a specific value to STK. Its centrality has been examined through many different theories or methodological frameworks such as relevance theory, acts of speech or politeness studies. As a result, it has been assigned a series of specific functions: social and cultural implications, identity constructions, etc…

Just as we have mentioned, in the institutional context within which we are working, the general structure of the medical interaction in a consultation follows a series of sections. These sections are associated with specific linguistic resources, such as asymmetric conversational turn-taking and the use of precise linguistic structures.

This turn-taking in the analysis of institutional conversation is also characterized by asymmetries or differences in the doctor/patient power relationships. Heritage (1997: 175) mentions several types of asymmetry, but in that case the interventions are not associated with specific roles, social norms or well-defined tasks of the institutions in question, which is what occurs in the doctor-patient interaction.

Time is also an important factor in the general structure of the Spanish consultation for several reasons; the Spanish healthcare system is a universal system. All Spaniards, non-Spanish citizens below 16 years of age and pregnant women have the right to use this system. Inside this system, each doctor is assigned a certain number of patients. Patients are able to choose their primary physician, as long as that doctor's patient roster is not full or they have the express authorization of the doctor. On the other hand, the administration believes that the time devoted to each patient for a general consultation should be between 6-8 minutes. This is often criticized by the healthcare professionals themselves, especially when it involves people who do not know the language or the inner-workings of the institution, a situation which has become quite common in the last decade in Spain.

These characteristics might lead us to think that this time is spent "getting to the point" (focusing on the topic at hand), and that there would hardly be room for *small talk* (STK). However, just as Coupland (2000: 6) points out, institutional speech implies a dialectic between the speech itself and the social conventions that are part of that type of interaction. They are two inseparable elements brought together by the STK, which plays a role beyond merely keeping the conversation going.

Box 6.2.

> "Small talk cannot be segregated from the 'mainstream' concerns of talk at work. It is an intrinsic part of the talk at work complex" (Coupland 2002: 6).

Box 6.3.

> "It is not generally possible to parcel out meaning in neat packages of referential on the one hand and social or affective on the other. Talk is inherently multifunctional" (Holmes 2000: 34).

In the medical consultation, as an example of institutional speech, *small talk* occurs as in other institutional discourse (ID) settings; this talk is used strategically and has meaning, as the following example illustrates:

Box 6.4.

Example 1: (D= doctor, P= patient; P is a regular Spanish patient who suffers from cancer and who has come for a routine check-up)

1 P: Buenos días. *[Good morning]*

2 D: Hola, buenos días ¿qué tal?. *[Hello, good morning, how are you?]*

3 P: Bueno pues bien. *[Well, good.]*

4 D: ¿Qué tal va? ¿Cómo se encuentra?. *[How are you doing? How do you feel?]*

5 P: Normal, bastante. *[Normal, pretty normal]*

6 D: ¿Normal? Tiene muy buen color. *[Normal? Your color is very good.]*

This is the start of the consultation and we see the typical greetings used to initiate the conversation. However, in this case, it is not just a simple greeting but rather, the doctor, by using the routine phrase "¿Qué tal?"/How are you?, is in fact also asking the patient about her state of health, thus adding an informative function to the phatic function and placing this intervention in the patient assessment section. At this point, however, let's take it section by section and follow the consultation as previously outlined.

6.3.1. Initial greetings

The analysis of our corpus reveals that in this section, the usual routine phrases tend be used such as *buenos días/good morning, buenas tardes/good afternoon, hola/hello, ¿qué tal?/How are you?,* just as in example 2 below. This is especially true when the patient is not a regular patient. In these cases, after the greetings, it is usually the doctor who moves on to the next section, taking control of the conversation and asking the patient the reason for the visit:

Box 6.5.

Example 2: (P, Spanish patient, in a routine consultation as a health clinic) 1 D: Hola ¿Qué tal? *[Hello, how are you?]* 2 P: Hola, bien. *[Hello, fine.]*

With regular patients we find that after the greetings, the conversation tends to get right to the point. This is what occurs in example 3, where the patient, after responding to the greeting, moves on to the next phase, adding information without waiting for the doctor to ask:

Box 6.6.

Example 3 (P, Spanish patient, in a health clinic with his primary doctor) 1 D: Hola, ¿qué tal? *[Hello, How are you?]* 2 P: Bien. Ya me llamaron de Madrid para..."cografía" o como se llame... *[Fine. They've already called me from Madrid for the "trasound" or whatever you call it...]* 3 D: Para la ecografía. *[For the ultrasound.]* 4 P: Sí, en Madrid. Y...y luego ¿qué voy a hacer? ¿voy a tener que pasar a otro médico del Val o qué? *[Yes, in Madrid. And...and then what am I going to do? Am I going to see another doctor from Val or what?]*

In regards to the second question we raised, that is, regarding the use of STK in medical consultations with foreign patients who do not have a good command of the language and / or culture, our analysis reveals interesting information, which is illustrated in the following explanations and example:

Box 6.7.

Example 4: (Moroccan patient who does not speak Spanish and is accompanied by her husband (F)) 1 D: ¿Son de Marruecos, no? *[You're from Morrocco, right?]* 2 F: Sí, sí. *[Yes, yes.]* 3 D: Bueno, pues ya nos olvidamos de esto… *[Well, let's forget about all that now…]* A ver <u>¿qué pasa? [</u>*Let's see, what's going on?]* 4 F: Sí, sí *[Yes, yes.]* 5 F: <u>Aquí estamos [</u>*Here we are]* 6 D: Está muy blanca. *[She's very pale.]* 7 P: Sí, قل لو فيا لحريق (dile que me duele) *[Yes, tell him that it hurt]*

The underlined expression "What's going on?" can play two different roles:

(a) Phatic function: To establish and maintain cordial or friendly relationships. In this case it is not interpreted as a question but rather a greeting that might be equivalent to "How are you?" and can be answered with the second underlined expression ("Here we are"). Both the question and answer lack informative meaning and content.
(b) Informative function: to ask about what is happening, about the reason or problem that brings the patient to the doctor. Here, the meaning is "What is the reason for the consultation?" In this case the person formulating the question does not expect a response such as "here we are", but rather seeks information or, in other words, propositional and not formulaic content.

In example 4 the doctor asks "What's going on" not with the intention of starting polite conversation but rather to ask a question. This is clear for the following reasons: Firstly, although there can be conversations of that type at the beginning of medical consultations, such greetings are typically part of the first section or movement of the standard medical consultation, which we have previously described as fulfilling a phatic function. Secondly, if we apply our knowledge of certain cultural components, such as the structure of the healthcare system or the time limits involved, it is understood that that step is simply a greeting in the doctor-patient interaction. Thirdly, here the statement "What's going on?" does not occur at the beginning of the conversation, but rather after several lines (two of which are included in the recording). And finally, because this statement comes after two discourse markers ("Bueno, pues ya nos olvidamos de esto"/*Well let's forget about that now* and "A ver"/*Let's see*), the first of which indicates a change of topic ("nos olvidamos de esto"/*Let's forget about that*) and the second suggesting an explanation. In other words, even if the initial lines could have been interpreted as trivial conversation, the time had come to get the crux of the consultation (for more information see Valero-Garcés y Taibi, 2004).

6.3.2. Goodbyes

Continuing with the same reasoning, Tannen (1984: 19-20) argues that among the many causes for misunderstandings is the homonym/pragmatic ambiguity (the use of the same expression for different purposes) and pragmatic synonym (paraphrasing or the use of different expressions for the same purpose). The potential problems for communication created by the homonym and synonym (both on a lexical and pragmatic level) can generally be avoided with the help of context. However, this is not always the case, especially when routine phrases are involved, which is what occurs in the previous examples (1-4) and in the examples below, which correspond to the section of the consultation in which goodbyes are said:

Box 6.8.

Example 5: (P, Spanish patient, in health center) 1 D.: ¿Vale? *[Okay]* 2 P: Vale. *[Okay]* 3 D.: Venga *[Alright then]*

In this case we can see a typical goodbye using the often seen expression "vale"/*okay* which in line 1 serves an informative function given that at this part of the consultation it is really the equivalent of asking the question "¿está todo claro?"/*is everything clear?* as if to ask "¿Te has enterado del tratamiento y de lo que debes hacer?"/*Have you understood about the treatment and what you should do?*. However, in other consultations it could mean: "¿te has enterado de todo?"/*Have you understood everything?* or "¿quieres preguntar algo más?"/*Do you want to ask anything else?* In other words, it is an element that takes on meaning according to the context. In line 02, "vale"/*okay* shows agreement with the doctor's question, as if to say "sí, está todo claro"/*yes, it's all clear* and in line 03 "venga"/*alright then* is like a simple "adiós"/*goodbye*.

Box 6.9.

Example 6: (F: Spanish father in a pediatric consultation for his baby's routine check-up) 1 D: En el centro de salud que sea su centro, cuando un mes el bebé le llevan bebé para que le programen las vacunas, vayan controlando al niño, ¿eh?. <u>Y nada más. Ya está. Está todo bien</u>. /*In whichever health clinic is your health clinic, when the baby is a month, take him there to get his vaccines scheduled, to have them continue to follow him.* 2 F: Vale. *[Okay]*

In example 6 we again see how the doctor uses a series of routine phrases to say goodbye. The person being spoken to responds with a simple "vale"/*okay,* which again can have two functions:

(a) Phatic function: a goodbye, equivalent to "adios"/*goodbye*
(b) Informative function: equivalent to "me he enterado"/*I've understood,* "O.K."/*Okay*

6.3.3. Assessment and discussions of patient's state

After the greetings, the next step in a standard consultation is to find out the reason the patient is there, so as to be able to investigate the situation before moving on to diagnosis and treatment. This is the point at which one of the characteristics of institutional speech, asymmetry, begins to appear.

There are studies (v. Drew y Heritage, 1992; Ainsworth-Vaughn, 1998) that show how the doctor exercises his power and controls the consultation using strategies such as: giving orders, showing agreement or asking direct questions, summarizing the situation or reformulating part of the other person's speech, which is what Holmes (2000) calls "doing power". In the same manner, it is the doctor who most often decides whether or not to use ST since, as Fairclough mentions (1989: 72), the person who occupies the position of power – the doctor in this case- is he who has the ability to decide whether to use ST or not. This fact, along with the increasingly more apparent tendency to strip away the formality from institutional speech and to "conversationalize" these types of encounters (Fairclough, 1995), leads us to assume that a greater percentage of ST is used to fulfill specific functions, such as reducing the distance of knowledge and of power relationships, facilitating conversation, reducing tension and smoothing out relationships by making the patient feel more comfortable talking about his illness or responding to the doctor's questions, which many times are viewed as very personal or taboo.

Such a hypothesis is confirmed in our analysis of the following examples, where the use of familiar language orients expressions towards positive politeness:

Box 6.10.

Example 7: (D: Doctor, N: Nurse, M: a Spanish mother in a pediatric consultation in a health clinic. The baby, 7 months old, has a cold)

1 D: ¿No le notas en la..., que el pis le huela mal? ¿Huele cómo siempre? *[You haven't noticed that the....that his pee smells bad? Does it smell like normal?]*

2 M: *Sí [Yes]*

3 D: *Sí [Yes]*

4 N: Estás gordito! Bien, voy a pesarte (dirigiéndose al bebé). A ver, sujétele un poquito (a la madre) *[You're a chubber! Okay, I'm going to weigh you (talking to baby). Let's see, hold him a little (to the mother)]*

5 D: ¿Come bien? *[Is he eating well?]*

6 M: Sí *[Yes]*

7 D: *(to the mother): Don't give him that right now (referring to the pacifier)*

8 D: A ver,¿qué le damos para que se entretenga? (cogiendo al niño). Sujete ahí (a la madre). *[Let's see, What can we give him to keep him busy? (picking up the baby). Hold him right here (to the mother*

9 D: ¡Qué bonito! (hablando del bebé) *[You're so cute! (talking to the baby)]*

10 D: A ver, Pilar (dirigiéndose a la enfermera). ¿Llegó el informe? *[Let's see, Pilar (speaking to the nurse). Has the report come]*

The pediatrician (D), a woman in this case, asks the mother questions about how the baby is doing. According to the usual protocol for pediatric consultations in Spain, if the baby is under one year of age, the baby will be weighed and measured whenever he/she is brought to the doctor, regardless of the official requirements in terms of what height and weight checks must be done at what time. In this case it is the nurse who performs this task and in line 4 we see how she uses a phrase with a diminutive, undoubtedly giving the consultation a warmer and more affectionate tone. The same thing happens in line 9 when the pediatrician speaks directly to the baby. However, we can also see that a certain distance is kept between the pediatrician and the mother of the baby, when the doctor uses the formal "you", "usted", when speaking to the mother. This is something which is repeated on other occasions in our corpus.

Box 6.11.

Example 8: (M: Spanish mother in a pediatric exam in the hospital emergency room, as she undresses her baby)
1 D: Me vas contando qué come. *Tell me what he eats.]*
2 M: Pues puré de verduras, pero no le gusta mucho, pescado y... fruta y no le gusta huevos tampoco... *[Well, pureed vegetables, but he doesn't like that a lot, fish and...fruit. He doesn't like eggs either. [...]*
3 D: ¿No quiere? ¿lo has intentado? *[He doesn't want them? Have you tried it?]*
4 M: Sí. *[Yes]*
5 D: ¿Le has cogido la yema, y le das un trocito de yema y no le gusta? Bueno, pues más tarde. *[You've taken the yoke and given him a tiny bit of the yoke and he doesn't like it? Okay, well later on then.]*
6 M: La primera vez ha comido un poquito... *[The first time he ate a little bit...]*
7 D: Pero luego ya no. Pues te esperas. Dejas pasar un tiempo y lo vuelves a intentar. ¿Y leche toma? (dirigiéndose al bebé) *[But after that he didn't. Well, you can wait. Let some time go by and then try again. Does he drink milk? (Talking to baby)]*
8 D: ¿Has vomitado, chiqui? *[Did you throw up, little one?]*

In example 8, the pediatrician tries to obtain information through the traditional question and answer structure, soliciting short answers. We can see that in this case, she addresses the mother using the familiar you/"tu", even providing the mother information while asking yes or no questions (3) and at one point she even says, ("Bueno, pues más tarde"/well, later on then), using what can only be a colloquial tone. She uses this tonc again in line 7 when she says "Pues te esperas. Dejas pasar un tiempo y lo vuelves a intentar"/*Well, wait then. Let some time go by and then try again.* This colloquial tone is further accentuated during the consultation when the doctor speaks directly to the baby, just as was done in the previous example, using an affectionate term, "chiqui"/*little one,* as she waits for the mother to answer the question, which the mother does, in order to complete the assessmentphase of the consultation.

6.3.4. Discussion and prescription of treatment and / or technical testing

Before moving forward, we should mention how difficult it is to classify the consultation into different sections, given that the limits which divide these sections are so imprecise. The same goes for classifying what is or is not *small talk*. In this case, just as we explained in the first few pages and as the reader will have by now ascertained, we believe STK to be everything in the medical consultation which is not related to providing specific information. In other words, we consider *small talk* to be the use of routine expressions and talk of personal issues which are not related to the issues typically discussed during the medical consultation. Having clarified this, we will now go on to look at some examples which we have classified within the diagnosis and treatment section of the consultation.

The analysis shows that the colloquial, familiar tone that we observed in the previous examples continues in the example below. Institutional discourse, being an activity that is performed before the general public, is also influenced by the societal norms and the rules of politeness which surround social activities. Since a service is being offered, positive politeness and using STK as another way to help bring the speakers together helps the doctor to do exactly that. Comments about the patient's appearance, the characteristics of treatment, improvement in health or how easy and convenient a certain test can be are all examples of positive politeness. We can see this in the following example:

Box 6.12.

Example 9: (In a health clinic during a pediatric consultation. The patient is a baby and the Spanish mother is the speaker)

1 D: En la ecografía que le han hecho, la última que le han hecho, eh sólo tiene un poquito afectado el riñón derecho. El izquierdo está bien, eh. El riñón derecho tiene un poquito más de dilatación que tenía y... pues le tendremos que hacer alguna prueba más de las que le hemos hecho. La prueba que le tenemos que hacer ahora es para ver si hay obstrucción o no la hay, eh. Todo en vistas de que el riñón no se acabe dañando, mmm. Estas pruebas no las hacemos aquí. Nos las hacen en Madrid, mmm [*In the ultrasound they did, the last one that they did on him, um the right kidney is just slightly affected, the left one is fine, okay. The right kidney is a little more dilated than before and...well, we'll have to do one more test in addition to the ones we've done. The test we have to do now is to see whether or not there is a blockage, okay. All this is so there won't be damage to the kidney, mmm. We don't do these tests here. They are done for us in Madrid, mmm*]

2 M: ¿En Madrid? *[In Madrid?]*

3 D: En Madrid en un hospital que se llama "Ruber Internacional", eh. ¿Dónde vivís? *[In Madrid in a hospital called "Ruber International",okay? Where do you live?]*

4 M: Aquí.*[Here.]*

5 D: Aquí en Guadalajara. Bueno, os pueden poner transporte. Os pueden llevar en ambulancia. Simplemente en el metro, ¡uy!, en el metro, en el tren y luego os lo pagan, lo que pasa es que es una lata, porque hay que hacer trámites, eh. Se puede hacer. *[Here in Guadalajara. Well, they can provide you with transportation. They can give you a ride in an ambulance. Or just on the subway, oh boy! on the subway, on the train and then they'll pay it for you. The thing is that it's a pain, because there's red tape, you know. It can be done.]*

We see how the doctor employs the same structures that we have already seen and that are part of positive politeness (use of tu/*you* and forms of *small talk* such as *eh/okay, mmm)* while explaining the treatment or tests that the patient must continue to have in light of the diagnosis they are able to provide. Personal comments are also added (5).

Box 6.13.

Example 10: (Treatment consultation for an older Spanish patient, who comes with her son for a check-up and to continue with treatment for cancer. The doctor explains the treatment that the patient will receive from then on and the cycles that remain and how they are scheduled.)

1 P: Es un martirio chino *[It's like torture]*

2 D: Ya queda menos, mujer, hay que pensar en eso. *[You don't have much farther to go dear, you've got to think of that]*

As Díaz Martínez (2002: 145) mentions, in this example taken from her study "la quimioterapia y sus efectos" / "Chemotherapy and its Effects", for the patient, the process of receiving one cycle after another of chemotherapy can feel like "torture", not just because of having to suffer through the side effects of treatment, but also because of the organized expectancy of knowing when treatments will occur over a period of several months. In this case, the doctor responds to the patient's protests by asking her to think of the process as a path ("Ya queda menos" / *You don't have much farther to go*, 2), so that the farther along she is, the less she has left ahead. In this way, the doctor comforts the patient and also asks her to view the process in a way that will minimize psychological suffering: a process that will get better. To accomplish this she employs the strategy of using STK, inserting a personal comment as well as a phatic marker, which in this case is "mujer" (literally, *woman*, but perhaps more comparable to how *girl* or *man* might be used in English in some circles).

Below there is an example in which the patient has limited knowledge of the language and hospital protocol.

Box 6.14.

Example 11: (Pediatric consultation, foreign patient)

1 D: Bueno, pues aquí se lo escribo, para que pueda alguien leérselo y decírselo para que se entere bien de todo, eh. *[Okay, well I'll write it down for you here, so that someone else can read it and tell you so that you understand everything well, alright.]*

2 P: Sí. [...] *[Yes]*

3 D: Ahora pide cita para que le hagan una ecografía y volver a hacerle la orina, el cultivo, eh. Esto es el volante y esto es el volante para el cultivo. Que le den para dentro de unos días, eh, como mucho dentro de un mes. *[Now you need to ask for an appointment for them to do an ultrasound on you and so they can do the urine again, the culture, okay. This is the slip and this is the slip for the culture.]*

4 P: [...]

5 D: la puerta de salida, pues hay un mostrador grande, con unas ventanillas, hay mucha gente, justamente ahí a la salida, [...]. Venga por aquí [...] (tras el examen físico, indicándole que vuelva a la silla) Déjelo, déjelo. No pasa nada. [...] (al tratar de recoger la sabanilla de la cama que se había movido) [...]. *[Downstairs, downstairs when...., at the exit, well there's a big counter with windows, there are a lot of people, right there at the entrance [...]. Come through here [...] (after the physical exam, indicating for him to sit back down in the chair). Forget about it, forget about it. It's no problem. [...] (when trying to pick up the small sheet from the bed that had moved) [...].]*

In this example we can see how the doctor tends to explain the treatment more carefully and he writes it down, trying to make sure that the patient understands him and repeating what he says or writing it down when necessary.

The use of sentence such as "¿Me entiende bien todo lo que digo?"/*Does everything I have said make sense?*, "¿Lo entiende bien?"/*Does that make sense?*, "¿Has entendido?"/*Do you understand?* "¿Sabes lo que es?"/*Do you know what that is?*, "¿Entiendes lo que digo?"/*Do* you get what I'm saying? "Un virus, ¿sabes lo que es?"/*a virus, do you know what that is?,* are repeated fairly often when doctors talk to foreign patients who do not have a good command of Spanish and could be considered STK according to a study by Cortés and Camacho (2005) of interactive markers in informal interactions.

Analysis shows that if someone belongs to another culture, this is an important factor to keep in mind when considering the use and function of STK. This is true for two reasons: because ST can be handled differently in different cultures; when the speaker does not have a good command of the cultural and/or linguistic systems of the language being used to communicate, misunderstandings can arise if other functions are attributed to STK. In relation to this, Holmes (2000: 56) notes that while STK is considered to be rather marginal and peripheral in western cultures, in eastern cultures it is just the opposite. Citing the Japanese culture as an example, Holmes explains that for the Japanese, language is highly formulaic and the system of politeness is much more elaborate. Knowing this, it stands to reason that the use of STK is also more habitual in these cultures and that it serves social purposes. The studies from Metge y Kinloch (1978), Metge (1986, 1995), Case (1988), Cushner y Brislin (1996) provide more information to this respect. In Spain, some studies focused on linguistic anthropology (v. Raga Gimeno, 2005) can serve as a foundation by which to understand this complex world of relationships.

All of this is made more evident in our analysis with respect to the remaining two sections of the consultation, which are interwoven throughout the other sections within the general structure of the consultation. We are referring to casual interjections, which are informal comments made about everyday life issues or topics and official procedures. At these moments, the doctor focuses on the problems the patient has beyond his or her medical problem. Thus, these interjections essentially fall somewhere in between institutional conversation and casual conversation.

Our analysis of the corpus indicates that STK is more prevalent in these sections and although it is used with both groups of patients, these interjections are more frequent in the case of the doctor – foreign patient. In the first group (doctor – Spanish patient), we have only found examples of casual interjections in those cases where there seems to be a certain level of familiarity between the speakers, for example in the case of a doctor who has been a patient's primary doctor for a long time, a patient who goes to the doctor often, long treatments and chronic diseases which require periodic visits. These are factors that influence the frequency with which this type of communication is used. Let's begin with the casual interjections.

6.3.5. Casual interjections

For centuries, western medicine has focused on medicine itself, and has not taken the patient's other needs, such as social and psychological needs, into account. It wasn't until the 1990's that a movement towards a more psychosocial model of medicine came about (v. Sharf, 1988; Deber, 1994; Steward, Gold y McDowell, 1995). The special edition of the publication *Health Communication* in 1997 entitled "The Patient as a Central Construct in Health Communication Research" is evidence of this, although there are some previous examples in articles published in 1973 in *The Journal of Communication*. In that issue different authors advocate for developing a closer relationship with the patient with the goal of reducing the imbalance that exists between doctor and patient and to help improve relationships and outcomes in medicine, as some previous studies had already demonstrated (Thompson, 1994; Heszen-Klemens y Lapkinska, 1984; Kaplan, Greenfield y Ware 1989; King, 1991). The results of these research studies indicated that cultivating interpersonal relationships in the medical consultation boosted the level of satisfaction patients had with their medical care. This played a role (or could play a role) in the decline in the number of reports filed for malpractice and in improved outcomes in medical consultations, compliance with treatment and helping to facilitate testing. One way to attain this type of relationship, one that goes beyond what is merely instrumental, is through the use of *small talk*.

That said, in our corpus we have found some differences in the relationship between health care professionals and non-Spanish patients in the sense that the doctor seems more inclined to provide extramedical information or information about official procedures – as we have observed in previous examples which included STK. This supports Ragan's (2000) assertion that the interactions that take place in healthcare centers are models of an emerging social construction and not static situations dependant on the role that each participant must play (doctor – patient). On the contrary, in these interactions the participants play with the language in order to mutually facilitate the social and medical task that each encounter holds:

Box 6.15.

Through discourse that otherwise might be labelled insignificant or at best peripheral to the alleged, superordinate medical goals of interview, diagnosis, examination, and treatment- that is, the discourse relational communication or 'small talk'- the profound asymmetry of the provider-patient encounter can be mediated. (Ragan 2000: 273).

In one of the examples that were discussed previously, example 9, we see how the pediatrician, after telling the patient that they have to do some tests in another city (41), adds a personal comment ("lo que pasa es que es una lata"/*the thing is is that it's a pain*), expressing her opinion and steering the patient in her choice between one of two options: going by ambulance or going on her own using public transportation.

These types of interjections are even more common in the case of foreign patients:

Box 6.16.

Example 12: (Doctor and Bulgarian patient in a health clinic. The patient has a bone condition and the doctor has prescribed pills and has also discussed that it is good to follow a diet rich in calcium).

[…]

1 P: Una bolsa [Silencio]/*a bag [Silence]*

2 P: y yo comprar queso […] y comer/*and I to buy cheese […] and to eat*

3 D: ¿Sí? ¿Queso? Eso es bueno para el hueso./*Alright? Cheese? It's good for the bone.*

Having completed the treatment phase, in line 1 the patient interrupts the silence by simply saying "Una bolsa"/*a bag,* while the doctor writes the prescriptions for the medicines the patient needs to purchase and take. The patient doesn't obtain a good answer because the doctor does not know the patient is talking to him (a woman was with the patient), perhaps because he hasn't understood well or because he doesn't want to listen. The patient persists, providing more precise information: "y yo comprar queso … y comer"/*and I to buy cheese and to eat*, and the doctor reacts with a "sí" / *alright?* a *small talk* formula indicating that he has listened as he adds a comment (which reinforces his interest in the patient and his problems).

In example 13, we again find a casual interjection from the patient, who brings up a personal issue:

Box 6.17.

Example 13: (Moroccan patient talks about his father while the doctor writes up the patient's treatment)

1 P: Cuando él ha venido en aquí, yo le he arreglado todo. La ha dejado los papeles para comisaría. Para... una residencia de cinco años, entra, sale, de todo. Pero, como es tan nervioso está muy mal, no aguanta mucho aquí, y al verano, se dijo tengo que ir, tengo que ir. Bueno. *[When he came in here, I had arranged everything for him. I had left him the papers for police department. For…a five year residency, he comes in, he leaves, everything. But, since he is so nervous, he is in really bad shape, he doesn't last long here and in the summer, he said to himself I have to go, I have to go. Well.]*

2 D: Dos, hacemos dos de....*[Two, we'll do two of...]*

3 P: Hace un favor si es posible sí. Que como ha venido aquí, no hay familias, no hay amigos. Todo el día está solito en la casa, como dice está un poquito *[You do me a favor if it's posible, yes. Since he has come here, there are no families, no friends. All day he's all alone at home, like you said he's a little.]*

4 D: Y no habla español. *[And he doesn't speak Spanish.]*

5 P: No habla español, ni nada. Y sabes una cosa, de nuestra conquista, todo el día con la mi mujer. Y a mi mujer no, no dice nada con él. *Na* más que hola, y buenos días y *na* más. Respeto de los abuelos *era* así. Hola y buenos días. Nada. Nada. *[He doesn't speak Spanish or anything. And you know something, about our conquest, all day with the my wife. And my wife doesn't doesn't say anything with him. Just hello and good morning and nothing else. Respect of the grandparents was like that. Hellos and good morning. Nothing. Nothing.]*

6 D: No, no. *[No, no.]*

7 P: Ni sienta con ellos, ni ver la televisión con ellos, ni nada, de nada. *Na* más que dan de comida y *na* más. *[No sitting with them, no watching television with them, nothing at all. Nothing more than they feed them and nothing else.]*

8 D: Ahh. *[Vale.]*

The inclusion of this interjection –just as in other examples we have encountered– is not considered to be "unprofessional" or inappropriate, but rather, on the contrary, it seems to promote good relations and the doctor listens and even participates in the conversation by adding information (4) (see Díaz Martínez 2002) , but also lets the patient speak.

6.3.6. Official procedures

With respect to the section on official procedures, these interruptions also constitute STK to the extent that it is not information which is directly related to the consultation and which adds another dimension to the role of the doctor in institutional discourse. As Díaz Martínez (2002: 40) indicates, the Spanish health care system makes the patient the central component in managing his own problems, since he must go from one department to another with prescriptions and referral slips and must figure out the procedure to follow in each department and which department is the right one. His success will depend on his ability to follow these steps in the best possible manner and in the least amount of time. This will require solid knowledge not just of the language, but also of the whole institutional system, something which the majority of migrant patients that go to medical consultations do not possess. We believe that this is the reason why these interjections are more common in consultations involving foreign patients.

In order to guide/help the patients, the doctor devotes a portion of the appointment to providing the patients with explanations and information about how to follow these formal steps and procedures: how to request an appointment in another clinic, how to get there, how to find out where to get tests done, providing information about the nearest pharmacy, etc. To provide the patient with this information, the doctor sometimes makes use of routine phrases, a colloquial tone or adapts his language to the patient. The goal is to make the patient feel more comfortable or to reduce the asymmetry we have already discussed and to lend a colloquial tone to the conversation, as example 14 demonstrates:

Box 6.18.

Example 14: (Health clinic. The doctor asks the patient for his appointment card, a card that all patients must have for appointments with the specialist)

1 D: ¿Y no le dio...? ¿no le dieron un cartón pequeño.. un papelito donde le apuntaban las citas que usted tenía? *[And they didn't give it to you...? They didn't give you a little cardboard...a piece of paper with the appointments you had written down?]*

2 P: Sí... me parece que... *[Yes...I think that...]*

3 D: ¿Lo tiene en casa? *[Do you have it at home?]*

4 P: Sí. *[Yes.]*

5 D: Pues con ese cartón puede ir al Val y pedir cita para recoger las pruebas que le han hecho. *[Well with that card you can come here to Val and request an appointment to get the results for the tests you've had done.]*

6 P: Aaaah *[Aaaah]*

7 D: ¿Vale? *[Okay?]*

8 P: Vale, sí. *[Okay, yes.]*

9 D: Cuando le hagan todo esto el cardiólogo le va a hacer un informe *[Once they do all that the cardiologist is going to send you a report]*

10 P: Sí. *[Okay.]*

11 D: Sí, para saber como está... *[Right, so you know how...]*

12 P: con estos sobres, entregar... *[with these envelopes, deliver...]*

13 D: Entonces, con ese informe es cuando vamos a proponerle para una invalidez. *[Then, once we have that report, that's when we can apply for for disability for you.]*

14 P:Sí. *[Yes.]*

15 D: Para que le declaren incapacitada para trabajar.... pero yo prefiero... por eso se lo decía, prefiero esperar a que termine bien todo el estudio, para tener bien todas las pruebas y todo eso para presentarlo en el tribunal. *[So that they'll declare you disabled and unable to work...but I prefer....that's why I was telling you, I prefer to wait in order to finish the entire study properly, to have all the tests right and all that to be able to present it to the court.]*

16 P: Sí, sí, vale. *[Right, right, Okay.]*

The doctor gives additional explanation using a colloquial tone, lending more emotion and warmth to the conversation. The participants themselves are the ones who regulate their use of STK, which are not fragments or exchanges devoid of meaning and which do not have a set place in the conversational structure.

Movement from one strategy to another to usually done in a manner which is both subtle and appropriate. This is especially true in the case of the professional, whose superior knowledge of the language allows him a greater command of the use of colloquial speech as well. This can even lead the professional to speak with grammatical error as part of this process of "colloquialness" in institutional discourse that Fairclough (1995) indicates. Example 15 illustrates this:

Box 6.19.

Example 15: (In the healthcare center. Foreign patient with minimal knowledge of Spanish. The doctor is trying to explain how to follow treatment. On a piece of paper he has drawn something that he shows the patient as he speaks.)

1 D: Noche no tomar, sólo por la mañana ¿vale? Mira esto [le enseña un dibujo]. El domingo, este trozo y este trozo que has guardado te lo tomas ¿eh? Así todos los días… Vamos a bajar poco a poco./*Night no take, only in the morning, okay? [Look at this [he shows him a drawing]. Sunday, this bit and this bit that you have set aside you take them, okay? Like that every day.]*

6.4. Conclusions

Just as it does in everyday conversation, *small talk* serves several functions in institutional discourse. In the specific case of the medical consultation, our study reveals that STK is used throughout the different sections which make up the general structure of the medical interview.

Likewise, we have confirmed the difficulty that lies in categorizing the different functions of STK, which are varied, and how challenging it is to separate what is STK from what is not and to distinguish the different sections of the medical consultation. The divisions are imprecise in both cases.

A conversation is a complex network of relationships and it is thus difficult to provide a general classification of the function(s) of each separate part of speech. As a whole we have ascertained how the use of STK serves different functions depending on the speaker, place and time that it is used within the general structure of the medical consultation. The most common of these functions are: keeping the conversation going or showing that he/she is following the conversation, softening the distance by using positive politeness, promoting the doctor-patient relationship by showing trust, alleviating anxiety or fear about a test, result or diagnosis, making clear the need to continue treatment, comforting the patient and helping to improve the patient's mood.

The general conclusion is that these functions go beyond just the phatic function. This is accentuated even more in the case of the doctor – foreign patient who does not have a good command of the language or the context of the workings of the Spanish health care system. In this case, the colloquialness of the conversation is accentuated and the use of STK by both parties is heightened, with casual interjections and explanations of official procedures reinforced by the use of interactive markers that serve as *small talk*, for example "¿me entiendes?" / *Does that make sense?*, "Sí?" / *Yes*.

We are aware of the fact more in-depth research is needed, with more extensive corpora that would allow for more general conclusions and a deeper exploration of some of the topics we have suggested or addressed here. Nevertheless, this study has provided a glimpse of the value of context and the great influence of extralinguistic elements which, in our specific context, might be, for example, the urgency of the task (due to time limits in the Spanish health care system), the personal relationships between speakers (regular or new patients), the cultural origin (lack of knowledge about customs) or command of the language (foreign users with trouble communicating). All of this can play a part in eliminating or increasing the use of emotional or social expressions and the use of STK. STK is not void of meaning and likewise, cannot be studied in a void.

Practice

This section contains activities to reinforce the information provided in the previous section. The activities can be grouped into two main types: activities for reflection and assimilation of content and activities directed towards research, implementation of skills and strategies in multilingual settings. These activities can be undertaken individually, in pairs or small groups and / or with people from different cultural backgrounds to provide fertile grounds for discussion in class or via email. This will depend largely on the way the book is used (e.g. for self-study, as a textbook, or as support material for any course connected with intercultural communication).

Activity 1.

After having read the chapter, answer the following questions:

1. How would you define *small talk*?

2. Do you think STK has a merely phatic function?

3. What factors do you feel influence the use of STK?

Activity 2.

Reflection. Think about your behavior during a medical consultation – both as medical professional and patient – and comment on what you do in relation to the use of *small talk.*

Activity 3.

Think about or observe conversations during consultations and copy down examples of *small talk.*

Activity 4.

Translate into your own language the following conversation. Identify examples of *small talk*, and write a comment about their meaning /functions in the text.

N = Nurse, P= Patient

N: So, it's time to discharge you home from the emergency room.

P: Great!

N: I have your discharge instructions here. You came in because of an infected wound on your toe.

P: That's right.

N: The doctors involved in your care were Dr. Allen and Dr. Marks. These are the medications you are going home on. The doctors have prescribed you an antibiotic for your infection. It needs to be taken for once a day for 10 days. Even if you start to feel better, you must finish the whole course of antibiotics – that is very important.

P: Okay

N: You have no restrictions, but you should take it easy for the rest of the day. Things to watch for would be if the wound becomes more red, if any pus or yellow discharge comes out of the wound, it you develop red streaking of the skin or fever. If any of that occurs, you should come back to the hospital.

P: Am I able to work?

N: That depends, what do you do for work?

P: I am a secretary.

N: That should be fine. You can return tomorrow. I will write a note excusing you for today. Do you have any questions?

P: Yes, do I need to do any follow-up?

N: Good question. You can remove the bandage yourself in three days. After that, leave the wound open to air as much as possible. Make an appointment with your PCP for 1 week from now. Any more questions?

P: No, that was it.

N: Okay, sign here and you are good to go.

Notes

* A preliminary version of this paper was published in Spanish in *Oralia,* 2008, Vol. 11, 107- 131 under the title "La conversación de contacto en encuentros institucionales: la consulta médica".

Bibliographical references and further reading

Ainsworth-Vaughn, N. (1998). *Claiming Power in Doctor-Patient Talk.* New York Oxford University Press.

Atkinson, P. (1999). "Medical discourse, evidentiality and the construction of professional responsibility". In Sarangi, S. and Roberts, C. (Eds.)

Talk, Work, and Institutional Order: Discourse in Medical, Mediation and Management Settings. New York: Mouton de Gruyter, 75-106

Borrell, F. (2004). *Entrevista clínica. Manual de estrategias prácticas*. Barcelona: SEMFYC.

Candlin, C. (2000). "General editor's preface". In Coupland, J. (Ed.) *Small Talk*. London: Longman, 13-20.

Case, S. (1988). "Cultural differences not deficiencies: an analysis of managerial women's language". In Rose, S. and Harwood, L. (Eds.) *Women's Careers: Pathways and Pitfalls*. New York: Praeger, 41-63.

Cicourel, A. (1992). "The interpenetration of communicative contexts: Examples from medical encounters". In Goodwin, C. and Duranti, A. (Eds.) *Rethinking Context*. Cambridge: Cambridge University Press, 291-310.

—. (1995). "Medical speech events as resources for inferring differences inexpert-novice diagnostic reasoning". In Quasthoff, U.M. (Ed.) *Aspects of Oral Communication*. Berlin: Walter de Gruyter, 364-387.

Conley, J.M. and O'Barr, W.M. (1990). *Rules versus Relationships: The Ethnography of Legal Discourse*. Chicago: University of Chicago Press.

Cortes, L. and Camacho, M. M. (2005). *Unidades de Segmentación y Marcadores del Discurso*. Madrid: Arco/Libros.

Coupland, J. (2003). "Small talk: social functions". *Research on Language and Social Interaction*, 36, 1-6.

Coupland, J. (Ed.) (2000). *Small Talk*. London: Longman.

Coupland, J., Coupland, N., and Robinson, J.D. (1992). "'How Are You?': Negotiating phatic communion". *Language in Society*, 21, 207-230.

Coupland, N. and Ylänne-McEwen, V. (2000). "Talk about the weather: small talk, leisure talk and the travel industry". In Coupland, J. (Ed.) *Small Talk*. London: Longman, 163-182.

Coupland, N., Wiemann, J.M. and Giles, H.N. (1991). "Talk as 'problem' and communication as 'miscommunication': an integrative analysis". In Coupland, N., Giles, H.N. and Wiemann, J.M. (Eds.) *"Miscommunication" and Problematic Talk*. Newbury Park, London and New Delhi: Sage, 1-17.

Cushner, K. and Brislin, R.W. (1996). *Intercultural Interactions. A Practical Guide*. London: Sage.

Deber, R.B. (1994). "The patient-physician partnership: Decision making solving and the desire to participate". *Canadian Medical Association Journal*, 423-427.

Díaz Martínez, F. (1999). "Asimetría profesional en la consulta de oncología: algunas constricciones conversacionales de la clínica". *Discurso y Sociedad*, 1(4), 35-68.

—. (2002). "La quimioterapia y sus efectos". In González Barón, M., Díaz Martínez, F. and Ordoñez Gallego, A. (Eds.) *La Relación Médico-Paciente. Una Visión Sociológica.* Barcelona: Ars Medica, 141-158.

Drew, P. and Sorjonen, M.L. (1997). "Institutional dialogue". In Van Dijk, T.A. (Ed.) *Discourse as Social Interaction,* London, Sage, 92-118.

Drew, P. and Heritage, J. (Eds.) (1992). *Talk at Work.* Cambridge: Cambridge University Press.

Fairclough, N. (1989). *Language and Power.* London: Longman.

—. (1995). *Critical Discourse Analysis.* London: Longman.

Fisher, S. and Todd, A.D. (Eds.) (1993). *The Social Organization of Doctor-Patient Communication* (2nd ed.). Norwood, NJ: Ablex.

Heritage, J. (1997). "Conversation Analysis and Institutional Talk". In Silverman, D. (Ed.) *Qualitative Research: Theory, Method and Practice*. London: Sage, 161-182.

Heszen-Klemens, I. and Lapinkska, E. (1984). "Doctor-patient interaction, patients health behaviour and effects of treatment". *Social Science and Medicine,* 19, 9-18.

Holmes, J. (2000). "Doing collegiality and keeping control at work: small talk in government departments". In Coupland, J. (Ed.). *Small Talk.* London: Longman, 34-61.

Kapland, S.H., Greenfield, S. and Ware, J.E. (1989). "Impact of the doctor-patient relationship on the outcomes of chronic disease". In Steward, M. and Roter, R. (Eds.) *Communicating with Medical Patients*. Newbury Park, CA: Sage, 28-235.

King, P.E. (1991). "Communication, anxiety, and the management of postoperative pain". *Health Communication,* 3, 127-138.

Long, A. (1983). "Linguistic and conversational adjustments to non-native speakers". *Studies in Second Language Acquisition* 5(2), 177-193.

Maynard, D.W. (1991). "On the interactional and institutional bases of asymmetry in clinical discourse". *American Journal of Sociology,* 92, 448-95.

Metge, J. (1986). *In and Out of the Touch: Whakamaa in Cross-Cultural Context.* Wellington: Victoria University Press.

—. (1995). *New Growth from Old. Whaanau in the Modern World.* Wellington: Victoria University Press.

Metge, J. and Kinloch, P. (1978). *Talking Past Each Other: Problems of Cross-Cultural Communication.* Wellington: Victoria University Press/Price Milburn.

Mishler, E.G. (1994). "The struggle between the voice of medicine and the voice of the lifeworld". In Conrad, P. and Kern, R. (Eds.) *The Sociology of Health and Illness: Critical Perspectives*. New York: St. Martin's, 288-300.

Raga Gimeno, F. (2005). "Médicos, marabouts y mediadores: Problemas de comunicación intercultural en la atención sanitaria a los inmigrantes de origen senegalés". In Valero-Garcés, C. (Ed.) *Traducción como Mediación Entre Lenguas y Culturas / Translation as Mediation or How to Bridge Linguistic and Cultural Gaps.* Alcalá de Henares: Servicio de Publicaciones de la Universidad.

Ragan, S. L. (2000). "Sociable talk in women's health care contexts: two forms of non-medical talk". In Coupland, J. (Ed.) *Small Talk*. London: Longman, 268-287.

Sarangi, S. and Roberts, C. (1999). *Talk, Work and Institutional Order*. Berlin: Mouton de Gruyter.

Schegloff, E. (1987). "The routine as achievement". *Human Studies*, 9, 111-151.

Sharf, B. F. (1988). "Teaching patients to speak up: Past and future trends". *Patients Education and Counselling* 11, 95-108.

Steward, R.L.Jr., Gold, W. R. and Mcdowell, T. (1995). "Discussing health related quality life in parental consultations". In Morris, G.H. and Chenail, R.J. (Eds.) *The Tasks in the Clinic: Explorations in the Analysis of Medical and Therapeutic Discourse*. Hillsdale, NJ: Erlbaum, 209-231.

Tannen, D. (1984). *Conversational Style: Analyzing Talk Among Friends.* Norwood, NJ: Ablex.

Thompson, T. L. (1994). "Interpersonal communication and health care". In Knapp, M. and Miller, G.R. (Eds.), *Handbook of Interpersonal Communication*. Thousands Oaks, CA: Sage, 696-725.

Tzanne, A. (2000). *Talking at Cross-Purposes,* Amsterdam/Philadelphia, John Benjamins.

Valero-Garcés, C. (2002a). "Análisis conversacional de las interacciones entre proveedores de servicios y usuarios inmigrantes en los centros de salud". *Oralia,* 5, 265-296.

—. (2002b). "Modificaciones en la conversación institucional. Análisis de los turnos de habla en la entrevista clínica con pacientes inmigrantes". In Luque, G. (Ed.) *Las Lenguas en un Mundo Global*. Jaén: Servicio de Publicaciones de la Universidad de Jaén, 29-38.

Valero-Garcés, C. and Taibi, M. (2004). "Análisis de la interacción comunicativa en contextos institucionales entre proveedores de servicios, usuarios e intermediarios lingüísticos". *Oralia,* 7, 173-194.

West, C. (1990). "Not just doctor's orders". *Discourse & Society* 1(1), 85-112.

—. (1993). "'Ask me no questions': An Analysis of queries and replies in physician-patient dialogues". In Todd, A.D. and Fisher, S. (Eds.) *The Social Organization of Doctor – Patient Communication*. Norwood, NJ: Ablex, 127-157.

CHAPTER SEVEN

RAPPORT MANAGEMENT STRATEGIES IN INTERCULTURAL MEDICAL ENCOUNTERS

Key Points

- Approaches to interpersonal relationship management
- Defining rapport management strategies
- Analyzing different types of encounters
- Variations in the strategies implemented when managing interpersonal relationships

Key Readings

Galanti, G.A. (2004). *Caring for Patients from Different Cultures*. Philadelphia, PA., University of Pennsylvania Press.

Raga Gimeno, F. (2008). *Mediaciones Interculturales*. Valencia, Universitat de València, Lynx.

Spencer-Oatey, H. (2008). (ed.). "Introduction". Helen Spencer-Oatey (Ed.), *Culturally Speaking: Culture, Communication and Politeness Theory*. 2º ed. 1-8. London, Continuum.

Spencer-Oatey, H. & Franklin, P. (2009). *Intercultural Interaction. A Multidisciplinary Approach to Intercultural Communication*. Basingstoke: Palgrave/Macmillan.

7.1. Introduction

This chapter might be considered an extension to the study presented in the previous chapter on the use of language in a specific institutional context: the medical encounter. The focus will be on *rapport management strategies* and the primary aim will be to present a comparative analysis of these strategies as they are used in two types of interactions: 1. Healthcare professional – Spanish patient; 2. Healthcare professional – non-Spanish-speakiong patient (NSSP).

7.2. Defining *rapport management strategies*

The starting point will be Spencer-Oatey and Peter Franklin's (2009: 102) definition of *rapport* and *rapport management:*

Box 7.1.

"We use 'rapport' to refer to people's subjective perceptions of (dis)harmony, smoothness-turbulence and warmth-antagonism in interpersonal relations, and we use the term 'rapport management' to refer to the ways in which this (dis)harmony is (mis)managed" (Spencer-Oatey and Franklin, 2009: 102)

In the previous chapter we analyzed the role of *small talk* in medical encounters and, specifically, those encounters involving foreign patients who do not have a thorough command of the language and/or knowledge of the workings of the Spanish healthcare system. Small talk is understood as the use of certain elements in a conversation which do not contribute any information directly to the topic at hand, but rather help keep the conversation going. The study revealed that certain problems arise during medical encounters between Spanish doctors and their foreign patients, who do not share the same norms of interaction.

A previous study (Valero-Garcés 2002) also confirmed that during these types of encounters with foreign patients, there were a greater percentage of incidental additions, such as small talk or explanations of bureaucratic procedures. This appears to be due to both linguistic and cultural problems in the sense that doctors and patients may have different expectations and may adhere to different social conventions. This can lead to modifications in the structure of the encounter and result in defective communication.

In the current study, while taking these indicators into account, I intend to delve further into a specific area of these interactions; what I call *rapport management strategies* or approaches to interpersonal relationship management. Following upon the work of Spencer Oatey (2008), these strategies or approaches will allow us to see how the conversation is oriented; how positive interaction is established, maintained or heightened.

7.3. Approaches to interpersonal relationship management

A research project about communication management strategies in medical encounters was conducted in Spain between 2004 and 2008, when the influx of foreign populations was significant. Data comes from the same corpus of recorded conversations used to analyzed small talk (Chapter 6).

The complete corpus consists of seventy fivedigitally recorded real-life conversations that took place in healthcare centers and hospitals in the central region of Spain between 2004 and 2008. These conversations have been divided into three groups:

1. Health care professional – Spanish patient
2. Health care professional – foreign patient communicating in Spanish
3. Health care professional – foreign patient that does not speak Spanish – companion to patient who acts as interpreter.

I should also point out the difficulties in obtaining these types of recordings, not only due to privacy issues but also because of the participants' initial reluctance to be recorded. Added to this is the almost total absence of professional interpreters in Spanish health clinics. In lieu of interpreters, this role must be filled by those who accompany patients to their appointments or by students completing internships as part of the Master's program in Intercultural Communication, Interpretation and Translation at the University of Alcala, Madrid. The conversations have been transcribed in the most straightforward way possible, focusing on content without duplicating special features such as pauses, silences, repeated sounds such as *ummm, ehhh…* The conversations were recorded by the doctors themselves, after obtaining permission from the patients and their companions. In this case I will be working exclusively with conversations from groups 1 and 2.

7.4. *Rapport management* strategies in medical encounters

When evaluating the type of *rapport management* strategies observed in this corpus of institutional conversations, it is worthwhile to also consider the conclusions drawn from the comparative study of these conversations. Specifically, it is useful to take into account other general aspects of these medical encounters, such as, an analysis of what occurs in each section of a standard medical consultation. Thus, in this chapter, we will be using information from the study presented in the previous chapter, adding comments about the rapport management strategies demonstrated in this type of institutional encounter.

7.4.1. Health care provider – Patient who speaks the same language

After the analysis of the conversations from group 1, the corpus -1. Healthcare professional – Spanish patient, and taking the previous research into account, the following are some of the results:

1. The doctor tries to follow the standard protocol for medical consultations by asking questions during the assessment phase and speaking for longer periods of time during the portion devoted to diagnosis and treatment, while the patient often speaks for longer periods of time in the sense that he / she provides more information than requested (2). This seems to contribute a more familiar tone to the conversation and creates a more relaxed atmosphere, elements which can be observed in example 1.

Box 7.2.

Example 1: Group 1 (D: Doctor; P: Regular patient; a woman around 60 years of age suffering from dizzy spells, who receives treatment)

1 D: ¿y se va encontrando mejor? ¿[va] teniendo menos mareos aunque de vez en [cuando como ayer?] *[Are you feeling better? [Are you] having less dizzy spells even if you do get them at times [like yesterday]?]*

2 P: [sí], [sí, en vez en cuando], pero no tanto como antes porque yo me iba como si estuviera borracha; me iba *pa* los *laos* y me tenía que agarrar pero estoy mejor. Ya solamente eso de así, de de la cabeza, a ver si voy a tener algo de la cabeza; ya le digo, (xxx) mi marido se acerca y él dice yo no te oigo nada, digo, bueno pero yo lo oigo, yo oigo una cosa así como muy lenta. Eso es lo que me tiene *quitao* a mi el sueño ¿eh? Porque mira, anoche, (xxx) esta pastilla esta que que me tomé, ésta es la que (xxx) y éstas me las mandó usted en una ocasión, pero que llevo ya tres noches que no duermo, anoche me tomé esa que ya me la había *tomao* a las once, y a las tres y media estaba sin dormir y tuve que echar mano a esta y ya me tomé dos, dos y nada; me dormí a las cinco y media; fue cuando me dormí, muy poco, y así que eso y otra vez que no sé si…*[[yes], [yes, sometimes], but not as much as before because it would be like I was going around drunk; I'd be swaying to one side and another and I'd have to grab on to something but I'm doing better. Now it's just the thing with, with with my head, we'll see if something is going on with my head; I'm telling you, (xxx) my husband gets closer up to me and he says I can't hear you at all, I say, but I hear it, I hear something like that like very slow. That's what's*

making me lose sleep, eh? Because look, last night (xxx) this pill this one that that I took, this is the one that (xxx) and these are the ones that you ordered for me on another occasion, but I haven't slept in three nights now, last night I took that one that I had already taken at eleven and at three thirty I still hadn't slept and I had to use this one and I took two, two and nothing; I fell asleep at five thirty; that was when I slept, very little, and so that was that and again I don't know if...]

3 D1: ¿Ha tenido sensación de que le giraran los objetos? ¿o no? *[Did you feel that things were spinning, or no?]*

4 P: Pues no. *[Well, no.]*

5 D1: ¿Qué le diera vueltas la habitación (xxx)? *[Like the room was spinning around you (xxx)?]*

6 P: No, lo único que (xxx) creo que eso es de la vista, que veo mucho a veces de este *lao*, pero vamos que yo creo que esto es.... *[No, the only thing (xxx) I think that it is due to my vision, that I see a lot sometimes on this side, but I think that this is...]*

2. *Small talk* is more common, especially when a regular patient is involved, which is true of several of the conversations in the corpus. This is partly due to how the Spanish healthcare system is organized. Given that each doctor is assigned a certain patient load and in this case, the recordings were all done by the same doctors. An example is presented below as means of illustration (14 – 18):

Box 7.3.

Example 2: Group 1 (D: Doctor; P: 60 year old patient with memory problems, at the end of the consultation)

1 D: ¿Cuándo decimos los médicos las cosas se las cree? *[When us doctors say things, do you believe them?]*

2 P: No, una… *[No, a...]*

3 D1: ¿o no se las cree? *[or don't you believe them?]*

4 P: Sí, señor, una se cree que los médicos unas veces aciertan o no aciertan, eso le pasa a todo el mundo igual. *[Yes sir, you think that sometimes doctors get it right and sometimes they don't get it right, that's the same for everyone.]*

5 D1: No le digo de acertar o no acertar, sino a si usted ve, [si le contamos] lo que hay. *[I'm not talking about being right or not being right, but rather if you see [if we tell you] what's going on.]*

6 P: Yo la verdad *[To tell the truth, I]*

7 D1: pues usted se va a ir a casa, y empieza a darle vueltas (xxx)

mañana *[Well you can go home and start thinking about it (xxx) tomorrow]*

8 P: No señor, estoy muy tranquila porque yo la verdad *[No sir, I'm feeling just fine but really I]*

9 D1: o a ver si va a tener un tumor o una cosa de esas *[What if you have a tumor or something like that]*

10 P: no, señor, yo la verdad desde que estoy con usted con (xxx) que me han *pasao* que con el primero lo he *pasao* muy mal y usted sabe que me ha *dao* unas pastillas y he ido muy bien y ahora también *[no, sir, really, since I've been seeing you, after all (xxx) that's happened, with the first one it was really bad and you know that you gave me some pills and things have gone well for me and now as well.]*

11 D1: mmm *[mmm]*

12 P: la verdad no puedo decir eso *[Truthfully I can't say that]*

13 D1: mmm *[mmm]*

14 P: mi hija se fue, porque dice que una vez, porque usted y mi marido estamos contentísimos, dice, es que yo estoy contenta con él pero es que me dio un día una contestación que no me sentó bien (xxx) *[my daughter left, because she says that one time, because you and my husband we're extremely happy, she says, the thing is, I'm happy with him but one day he answered me in a way I didn't like (xxx)]*

15 D1: *mmm[mmm]*

16 P: le dijo que le tomara la tensión y usted le contestó, le dijo a ver si se piensa que esto es un mercao *[She told you to take his blood pressure and you told her let's see here, do you think this is a store]*

17 D1: sí, algo así *[yes, something like that]*

18 P: y ella se (xxx) y por eso se fue, pero, la verdad, es que yo estoy contenta con usted *[and she (xxx) and that's why she left, but, the truth is I'm happy with you]*

19 D1: bueno *[well]*

20 P: la verdad, que sí, porque me ha pasado *[I really am, because I've been through]*

21 D1: bueno, ahora lo que vamos a hacer va a ser explorarle un poco *[well, now what we are going to do is examine you a little]*

22 P: sí *[yes]*

In this case we can see that a portion of the appointment is devoted to a discussion about the doctor and not about the patient's state of health.

3. Additionally, the more familiarity that exists between the speakers, the more small talk occurs, to the point where the patient can be the one who goes so far as to talk about issues more directly related to the doctor, as we saw in the previous example (14-16). This can also be observed in the example that follows (example 3):

Box 7.4.

Example 3: Group 1. (P: 70 year old patient with memory problems, when saying goodbye. There are two doctors present at the appointment, the attending doctor (D1) and a resident doctor who the patient refers to in the following example).

1 P: ¿que él se va a quedar con nosotros? ¿es el doctor este? *[Is he going to stay with us? Is this guy the doctor?]*

2 D1: no, él va a estar todo el año conmigo *[no, he is going to be with me the whole year]*

3 P: ah, es que creía .... *[ah, I thought...]*

4 D1: está haciendo la especialidad y está acabando este año la especialidad y va a estar aquí todo este año con nosotros y *[he's doing the specialty and is finishing the specialty this year and he's going to be here with us this year and]*

5 P: muy bien; es que pensaba que se iba usted y se quedaba él *[very well; I thought you were leaving and he was staying]*

6 D1: no, no, nos vamos *[no, no, come on now]*

7 P: muy bien *[very well]*

4. The percentage of filler words or other language-specific elements that are used is fairly high and certainly more varied in comparison to Type 2 encounters. The purpose is often keeping with what we understand by small talk: to make sure the person we are talking to is following us, to seek his approval or simply to make for a more friendly conversation. These are interventions such as: eh?/*eh?*, digo yo/*that's what I say*, ah/*ah*, vaya/wow, de acuerdo?/*alright?*, "Vale"/*okay*, "a ver"/*let's see*, "ummm"/*ummm*, as the previous examples confirm.
5. The greetings and farewells such as "buenos días"/*good morning*, "siéntese"/*have a seat*, "hasta luego"/*see you later* and "adiós"/*goodbye* are also more varied than in type 2 as are other

elements of small talk that play certain roles such as "vale"/*okay* or more individualized questions such as: "Virtudes, ¿qué le trae por aquí?"/*Virtudes, what brings you by?*, or even getting straight to the point, as in the following example:

Box 7.5.

Example 4: Group 1. (D: Doctor, P: Patient around 25 years old)
1 D1: ¿Qué tal vas de alpiste? *[How are doing with the meds?]*
2 P: bien *[good]*
3 D1: ¿y cuánto te ha durado? *[and how long have they lasted you?]*
4 P: bueno es que la última caja que me distes no tenía 15, era un mes *[well the last box you gave me didn't have 15, it was a month]*
5 D1: ¿un mes? *[a month?]*
6 P: 30 pastillas *[30 pills]*

In this case we can undoubtedly observe the familiarity with which the doctor treats the patient when he greets him with a question that requires an answer but also by using a colloquial expression to refer to the medication ("alpiste", literally, bird food).

6. The use of certain elements helps to positively orient the conversation and reinforces the interpersonal relationships, giving the medical encounter a more relaxed feel:
   a. Use of diminutives, especially in pediatric consults. For example: "cajita", literally, *little box"*, "¿alguna cosilla más?", literally, "*any other little thing?"*, "un pinchacillo"/*a little poke*, "dobla un poquito el brazo"/*bend your arm a little* "estás gordito"/*you are a little chubby,* "ovulito" / literally, *little egg*, "culete" / *tushy*.
   b. Doctor regularly refers to patient in "Usted" (formal "you" in Spanish) and by first name, for example, "Dígame, Carmen" / *"Tell me, Carmen*", "A ver, Claudia" / *"Let's see, Claudia",* "Jesús, ¿le duele aquí?" / *"Jesús, does it hurt here?",* "Vas a pasar aquí, María" / "*You're going to go here, Maria"....*
   c. Using "tú" (informal form of "you" in Spanish) with younger patients: "Te duele aquí"? / "*Does it hurt here?",* "¿Cómo te llamas? / *What's your name*"

7. Use of "nosotros"/we, by doctor especially in the diagnosis and treatment phases. This seems to serve several functions:
   a. Reaffirming that doctor belongs to an institution or group.
   b. The doctor feels supported by community.
   c. Reaffirms doctor's superiority to patient.
   d. Shows more camaraderie than using "I"

For example: "Le vamos a comentar..." / *We are going to talk about*, "y ahora le vamos a ver lo de la tensión"/*and now let's see about blood pressure*, "entonces vamos a hacer"/*So we're going to make...*" This is just what we see in the following example:

Box 7.6.

Example 5: Group 1. (D: Doctor, P: Patient: a woman of about 70 years of age with problems due to tension and anxiety, already in treatment) 1 D:[vamos a intentar] a ver si con una medicación conseguimos que se (xxx) solamente un *[[We're going to try] to see if we can get it to (xxx) just a little bit with medication]* 2 P: (xxx) 3 D: se le quiten los nervios y *[it calms your nerves and]* 4 P: y y el temblor que tengo de del pulso, que a veces me tengo que sujetar (xxx) con la mano *[and and the trembling I have in in my hand, sometimes I have to hold (xxx) with my other hand]* 5 D: eso lo veo normal [*I think that's normal]*

8. Using colloquial phrases that are signs of positive or friendly rapport management, for example, "comer el coco" (*to obsess over something or brainwash someone* literally, *to eat up the coconut),* "yo que sé"/*what do I know*, " que si patatín, patatán"/*and this, that and the other* to indicate that someone is going over an issue again and again:

Box 7.7.

Example 6: Group 1. (D1: Attending doctor; P: Spanish woman of about 60 years of age with memory problems) 1 P: y y, cuando subimos al pueblo cierra la puerta y empieza a decirle unas cosas a Julián, que luego ya bajando del pueblo, pues, y qué te ha dicho tu madre que ya te ha estado *comiendo el coco* para que vuelvas con ellos y no sé qué y no sé cuántos y *patatín y patatán* y brbrbrbrbr *[and,*

and, when we get up to town he closes the door and starts saying stuff to Julian and then when we were finally leaving town, well, and what has your mother told you, she's been brainwashing you so that you'll go back to them and so on and so forth and this that and the other and blah blah blah]

2 D1: mmm/*mmm*

3 P: y así/*and that's how it was*

4 D1: o sea que todavía sigues teniendo carencias en tu vida *[so you are still lacking things in your life]*

5 P: sí sí, y si y si hago algo mmm, por qué lo hago y mi hijo es mi hijo, y a mi es que me desquician muchísimo *[yes yes and if I do something, mmm, well I do it and my son is my son and the thing is, they really drive me off the deep end]*

These strategies help produce a relaxed, "coloquial" climate in the medical encounter. In the same sense signaled by Fairclough (1995), this shows the progressive colloquialism in institutional encounters, within which there is a desire to reinforce or maintain cordial relationships between speakers or, in Spencer-Oately's words (2009: 117): *rapport enhancement orientation* or "the desire to strengthen or enhance harmonious relations between the interlocutors.

7.4. 2. Health care professional – Migrant patient that speaks Spanish

Some of the results of the analysis of the second type of encounters show the following in comparison to the first type:

1. The doctor likewise tries to follow standard protocol for medical appointments, going through the different stages of the interview; however,
2. The doctor – and not the patient – is the one who tends to speak for longer periods, even during the assessment phase, asking questions that require a simple yes/no answer instead of asking open questions as in group 1. In this case, it is the doctor who tends to give the explanation and the patient is limited to monosyllabic or short phrase responses. The limits of language has various consequences – undoubtedly linked with a lack of competency in other aspects of rapport management such as: being unfamiliar with the institutional context (which in this case is healthcare); the speaker's lack of interest; lack of information; social distance or

influence due to emotional factors (Spencer Oatey 2009: 101). As a result, a feeling of even greater distance is created and one can even sense moments where the conversation actually seems to move away from a positive orientation and may become much less cordial.

The following example shows how a doctor goes about directing the conversation and constructing the interaction by dint of questions and by paraphrasing or repeating the patient's answer in an effort to maintain or reinforce the cordial doctor-patient relationship.

Box 7.8.

Example 7: Group 2. (P: 35 year old woman of Moroccan origin who has been in Spain for 5 years. Nature of consult: Hand that hurts and shakes)

1 D: ¿Qué pasó ayer? *[What happened yesterday?]*

2 P: Pues ayer están discutiendo mi (xxx) mi hermanos los dos eso sí *[Well yesterday my (xxx) my brothers are arguing, the both of them that's right]*

3 D: sus hermanos empezaron a discutir *[your brothers started arguing]*

4 P: sí *[yes]*

5 D: ¿y qué pasó? *[and what happened?]*

6 P: Pues me empezó mi mano así, me … *[Well my hand started like this, my]*

7 D: la mano *[your hand]*

8 P: sí *[yes]*

9 D: ¿pasó algo entre sus hermanos a parte de la de las voces o *[did something happen between your brothers apart from the vocally or]*

10 P: no *[no]*

11 D: nada más que se puso muy nerviosa al oírlos que que gritaban *[you just became very nervous hearing them yell]*

12 P: sí *[yes]*

13 D: y discutían entre ellos *[and argue amongst themselves]*

14 P: sí *[yes]*

15 D: vale, y desde entonces le tiembla la mano *[okay and since then your hand shakes]*

16 P: sí *[yes]*

17 D: ¿ha ido a más o a menos? *[has it gotten to be more or less?]*

18 P: más *[more]*

19 D: a más *[more]*

20 P: sí *[yes]*
21 D: ¿está nerviosa? *[are you nervous?]*
22 P: sí *[yes]*
23 D: sí ¿pero por algún motivo ya o ya está calmada por esa discusión? *[yes, but for some other reason or have you calmed down from the argument?]*
24 P: no estoy calmada ya *[I'm still not calm]*
25 D: sí, o sea que en teoría ahora no hay motivo aparente para que siga nerviosa *[right, so in theory there is now no apparent reason for you to continue being nervous]*
26 P: sí *[yes]*
27 D: ¿hay motivo? *[Is there is a reason?]*
28 P: no *[no]*
29 D: no pasa nada, no hay ninguna, no hay nin… ninguna circunstancia especial en su vida que haya ocurrido que le provoque estar nerviosa o preocupada por algo ¿hay algo que le preocupa? *[There's nothing going on, there's no... no special circumstance in your life that has happened to cause you to be nervous or worried about something. Is there something that worried you?]*
30 P: o sea mi enfermedad *[well my illness]*
31 D: lo de las manos *[the hand thing]*
32 P: sí *[yes]*

This clearly shows some of the common problems which have already been examined in other previously mentioned studies. These problems include the use of repetition with paraphrasing to ensure comprehension (23-25), where the doctor needs to speak up to 4 times in order to understand that the patient has no other reason for worry and that the patient has understood him or to look for confirmation from the patient (2-3) or to clarify something that is implicit (30-31). We can also observe the use of elements that help to transmit an air of trust, such as the use of fillers such as "no pasa nada"/*It's alright* and "vale"/*okay*.

3. The standard structure is modified when other sections are included, such as small talk or explanations of bureaucratic procedures. However, here it is the doctor who introduces these additional sections and not the patient, as was the case in Type 1. This is usually done in order to provide explanations regarding certain tests or treatments or things the doctor or patient must do, to explain aspects related to the customs of the country, to give advice about what might be done (calling an ambulance, applying for a health

care card, etc.) or to obtain additional information from the patient (where he/she is from, how long they have been in Spain). With respect to the latter point, questions to obtain more information can serve a dual function:

a. To help create a climate of confidence as part of the management of interpersonal relationships.
b. To obtain the information necessary to complete diagnosis by relating the patient's response with certain knowledge (for example, if they are from Morocco, thinking the child may not have been vaccinated for certain diseases.)

In this case, small talk is placed in that dual role of reference and transaction, something which we discussed in the 2008 study and in the collection of essays included by Placencia y García (2008) in Volume 11 of *Oralia,* which is devoted to the analysis of oral speech. Two examples follow:

Box 7.9.

Example 8: Group 2. (P: Moroccan woman and two children. Diagnosis: tuberculosis; to confirm this, doctor sends her for x-rays)

1 D: Ustedes van a calle Ferial *[You go to Ferial street]*
2 P: Aha *[aha]*
3 D: Con este papel *[With this paper]*
4 P: Aha *[aha]*
5 D: y le van a decir qué día tiene que ir para hacerse la placa. ¿Sabe lo que es la placa? *[and they're going to tell you what day you have to go get the film taken You know what the film is?*
6 P: ¿ah? *[ah]*
7 D: Una radiografía *[an x-ray]*
8 P: Vale *[Okay]*

Box 7.10.

Example 9: Group 2. (P: Romanian woman around 22 years old, with strong abdominal pain. A uterine cyst has been found)

1 D: Escúchame un momento. Tú no, no… si con los anticonceptivos no tienes suficiente no no se pueden tener tantos abortos *[Listen to me for a minute. You can't, can't...if with the birth control pills you don't have enough, there can't can't be so many abortions]*
2 P: Lo sé *[I know]*

3 D: y esos ..*[and those]*
4 P: No, que por eso [*No, because of that]*
5 D: y esos doce son abortos voluntarios que has querido hacerlos tú y eso no se
puede hacer o sea no te quiero decir porque yo no, no crea que se deba o no abortar sino que porque para ti y para tu propia salud…*[and those 12 are abortions that you wanted to have and that can't be, I mean, I don't mean to say it's because you should or shouldn't have abortions but rather for you and for your own health…]*
6 P: sí, no está bien *[yes, it's not okay]*
7 D: hay muchos métodos anticonceptivos hay DIUs hay más cosas ¿sabes? *[there are a lot of birth control methods there are IUDs there are more things, you know?]*
8 P: ¿y entonces qué hago? ¿pero la otra por qué no lo ha visto ese quiste? *[and so what do I do? But why didn't the other woman not see this cyst?]*
9 D: porque igual no estaba o no se vió *[because maybe it wasn't there or she didn't see it]*

In this case there is small talk. In line 1 the doctor takes on an almost paternal role, speaking to the patient in a very direct way as if to give her advice; and in line 2, he insists on making clear that what he is saying is for the patient's own good in order to avoid any misunderstanding due to personal issues. All of this is accompanied by other elements which help reinforce or develop friendly relationships: the use of the informal "you" ("escúchame"/*listen to me*), avoiding being overly direct so as not to appear imposing or wanting to exercise his role as doctor: ("tú no, no…"/*you can't, can't…*) and seeking out the most impersonal form ("no se pueden…."/*there can't be*), the search for balance and trying to justify his position, using fillers like "o sea"/*I mean*, "no te quiero decir"/*I don't mean to say*, avoiding using "nosotros"/*we* as an institution and preferring to use "yo"/*I*, which in this context brings him closer to the patient. The same goes for the filler that he uses to seek confirmation from the patient to find out if she is following him: "¿sabes?"/*you know?*

As for the patient, she used the simple phrase "la otra"/*the other one* to refer to another medical colleague, a reference that is inappropriate due to its pejorative nature. In this context, however, it demonstrates a lack of command in terms of the pragmatic use of the language.

4. The use of fillers or elements of small talk is greater than in Type 1; however, it is less varied, since the repetition of filler words such as "sí"/*yes* or "vale"/*okay* is more pronounced, as can be observed in the following example:

Box 7.11.

Example 10: Group 2 (D: Doctor; P: Moroccan patient diagnosed with tuberculosis)

D: y le van a decir qué día tiene que ir para hacerse la placa ¿sabe lo que es la placa? *[and they are going to tell you what day you have to go to get the film taken. Do you know what the film is?]*

1 D: ah? *[ah?]*

2 D: una radiografía *[an x-ray]*

3 P: vale *[okay]*

4 D: pero tiene que pedir la cita *[but you have to ask for an appointment]*

5 P: vale *[okay]*

6 D: ¿vale? *[okay]*

7 P: vale *[okay]*

8 D: ¿vale? Esto y esto *[okay? This and this.]*

9 P: vale *[okay]*

10 D: ala, nos vemos con los rayos y la placa *[alright, see you with the x-ray and the film]*

11 P: vale *[okay]*

12 D: adiós *[goodbye]*

13 P: adiós *[goodbye]*

5. The variety of greetings and goodbyes is reduced in relation to Type 1, generally limited here to the typical "buenos días"/*good morning*, "buenas tardes"/*good afternoon*, "hola"/*hello.* Sometimes, there is no greeting at all and the doctor instead jumps right into the appointment. Along these lines, we should mention that it is rather common that when the patient enters the room, the doctor is occupied writing up the previous patient's report or reading the history of the patient that is coming in or doing some other activity. In these cases, the patient tends to sit waiting until the doctor says something. Thus, there are sometimes several seconds of silence that seem to make a greeting unnecessary.

Misunderstandings can also occur when, for example, the greeting is confused for a question meant to obtain more information, just as is illustrated in the following example with the use of ¨Qué pasa?/*"What's going on?"*

Box 7.12.

Example 11: Group 2 (P: Moroccan patient who does not speak Spanish and who is accompanied by her husband (F) who is the one who speaks)
1 D: ¿Son de Marruecos, no? *[You're from Morrocco, right?]*
2 F: Sí, sí. *[es, yes.]*
3 D: Bueno, pues ya nos olvidamos de esto… A ver ¿qué pasa? *[Well, let's forget about all that now... Let's see, what's going on?]*
4 F: Sí, sí *[Yes, yes.]*
5 F: Aquí estamos *[Here we are]*
6 D: Está muy blanca. *[She's very pale.]*
7 P: Sí, قل لو فيا لحريق(dile que me duele) *[Yes, tell him that it hurts]*

"¿Qué pasa?"/*What's going on?"* can perform two different functions: phatic or informative, as we will explain below. In the first case, the intention is to establish or maintain a friendly and cordial relationship. In this case the expression should not be interpreted as a question but rather as a greeting and it is possible to respond with the other underlined expression ("aquí estamos"/*here we are*). Both the question and the answer are lacking in informational content or meaning.

In the case of the informative function, the intention is to ask about what is happening, about the reason or problem that brings the patient to the doctor. In this case the person asking the question does not expect a response such as "aquí estamos/*here we are*" but rather information or, in other words, prepositional and not formulaic content. (Valero-Garcés &Taibi 2004).

6. The relaxed climate of the appointment is similar to that of Type 1 in several aspects such as:
   a. The use of diminutives by the doctor – especially in pediatric consults. However, we should mention that the use of diminutives is even more pronounced in the case of patients of Latin-American origin: "pinchacito"/*little poke*, "doctorcito"/literally, *little doctor*.
   b. The doctor addresses the patients in a similar way, using the informal you ("tú") or formal you ("usted") (e.g..: "Iham, dígame que le pasa"/*Iham, tell me what's going on*, "A ver,

Mohamed"/*Let's see, Mohamed)*. Here, age seems to be the determining factor and the doctor addresses the patient as "tú" (informal you) or "nosotros" (we) in the case of younger patients ("Vas a pasar aquí, Claudia"/*you're going to come in here, Claudia*) just as in Type 1. Our analysis shows the doctor only resorts to using the first person when he/she seems irritated or tired of helping to keep the conversation going or when he wants to appear closer or more convincing to the patient. For example, when he says: "yo aquí le puedo dar esto, esto es el Valium, pero Valium tiene usted en su casa"/*here I can give you this, this is Valium, but you have Valium at home.* However, the type 2 patients address the doctor differently than the type 1 patients, something which seems to be more due to a lack of linguistic competence than to a pragmatic one. Some examples are:

c. The patient sometimes addresses the doctor in too direct a way by using the informal you "tú" in phrases such as "entiendes"?/*"Do you understand?"*, something that would not occur in the case of Spanish patients who usually prefer to use "usted". This difference can be seen in the following example.

Box 7.13.

Example 12: Group 2. (P: Bulgarian patient with foot pain) 1 P: sí, pero no, no me duele aquí ¿entiendes? Aquí a mi me duele el hueso ¿sabes? Cuando me hago masaje me deja y después otra vez cuando me levanto como si tengo ochenta años ¿sabes? Así me duele me pongo así/*Yes, but it doesn't, doesn't hurt me here, you understand? Here the bone hurts, you know? When I massage it it goes away and then it comes back again when I get up as if I was 80 years old, you know? It hurts like this I go like this.*

b. The use of words and expressions by the patient that are not typical in a peninsular Spanish speaker, causing the doctor to ask for repetition. This can even happen with Latin-American speakers and with the words and expressions they use. Another example of this, taken from the same conversation, can be found below:

Box 7.14.

Example 13: Group 2. (P: Bulgarian patient with foot pain)
1 D: ¿Dónde te duele? *[Where does it hurt?]*
2 P: aquí *[here]*
3 D: tienes ahí el dolor [dolor] y el dolor se te *[you have the pain (pain) here and the pain]*
4 P: tremendo *[terrific]*
5 D: ¿qué? *[what?]*
6 P: tremendo aquí digo que es tremendo mucho *[terrific here I mean it's a lot terrific]*
7 D: el dolor que es muy fuerte *[the pain is really bad]*
8 P: tremendo *[terrific]*
9 D: ¿y se te queda ahí localizado o se te va hacia algún sitio? *[and does it hurt only in one place or does it go somewhere else?]*
10 P: No me duele eso y la rodilla aquí después. *[No, that hurts and my knee here after.]*

In this case the doctor seems surprised by the patient's choice of words, which are uncommon in everyday speech and asks the patient to repeat what has been said. Another similar example is the use of the expression "Chiao, doctorcito"; literally, *Ciao, little doctor* by an Ecuadorian patient, an expression that would not be used by a speaker of peninsular Spanish.

c. Asking the doctor direct questions, something which is not typical among Spanish patients or foreigners who are not of Latin-American origin. The following example involves a variation in the standard structure of the medical appointment, given that the patient asks the doctor that he see her for something other than the original motive for the appointment, as we see below (4,6):

Box 7.15.

Example 14: Group 2 (D: Doctor, P: Ecuadorian patient in a gynecological check-up)
1 D: vas a pasar aquí Claudia. Te quitas el pantalón y la braguita *[You're going to come through here, Claudia. You'll take off your pants and underwear.]*
2 P: vale *[okay]*
3 D: Voy a explorarte y a hacerte otra vez la ecografía ¿vale? *[I'm going to examine you and do the ultrasound again, okay?]*

4 P: vale y después me hace alguien algo aquí por favor ¿la espalda me hace un control? *[okay and afterwards can't someone do something here please, can they check my back?]*
5 D: no sé lo que me (xxx) *[I don't know what (xxx)]*
6 P: por fa porque puedo *[please because I can]*
7 D: sí sí *[yes yes]*
8 P: aquí, me duele más o menos aquí, ahí ese ese es el punto vamos aquí no tengo nada ese *[here it pretty much hurts here, here that that is the spot, here I don't have anything]*
9 D: hay un dolor *[there's pain]*
10 P: ese/*[right]*
11 D: ¿y no te has [dado] *[and you haven't (hit) yourself?]*
12 P: [aquí] *[(here)]*
13 D: un golpe ahí ni nada? *[hit yourself there or anything?]*
14 P: no no yo tenía problemas por el riñón en pero hace dos años *[no no I had kidney problems in but that was two years ago]*

On the other hand, in the case of patients who come from other countries and who do not have good command of Spanish (Romanians, Polish, Bulgarians) monosyllabic responses such as "sí"/*yes* or "no"/*no* are common, even when something more is expected, as illustrated by the example below.

Box 7.16.

Example 15: Group 2 (D: Doctor, P: Bulgarian patient with muscle problems)
1 D: tiene que venir el lunes a citaciones; aquí pero allí donde la gente pide hora con este papel y este; bueno, con los dos, a que le den hora para el neurólogo ¿vale? Y tiene que ir al médico de cabecera a que le haga le receta, esto ¿vale? *[You have to come on Monday to the appointment desk; here but over there where people ask for an appointment with this paper and this; well, with both, so that they will give you an appointment to see the neurologist, okay? And you have to go to your PCP so that he'll write you the prescription, okay?]*
2 P: vale *[okay]*
3 D: yo aquí le puedo dar esto. Esto es el Valium, pero Valium tiene usted en su casa *[I can give you this here. This is Valium. but you have Valium at home]*
4 P: no *[no]*
5 D: ¿no? *[no?]*

6 P: tengo *[I have]*
7 D: ésta al desayuno y a la cena *[this one with breakfast and dinner]*
8 P: vale *[okay]*
9 D: por la mañana y por la noche *[in the morning and at night]*
10 P: vale *[okay]*
11 D: y esta por la noche sólo *[and this one just at night]*
12 P: vale *[okay]*
13 D: ¿vale? *[okay?]*
14 P: vale *[okay]*
15 D: sólo por la noche una al día de éstas *[only at night, one a day of these]*
16 P: vale *[okay]*
17 D: y esto para por la mañana y por la noche ¿vale? *[and this one for the morning and at night, okay?]*
18 P: vale *[okay]*
19 D: y tiene que ir con esto a su centro de salud y aquí a pedir hora para el neurólogo ¿vale? *[and you have to go with this to your health clinic and ask for an appointment with the neurologist]*
20 P: vale *[okay]*
21 D: no sé si se habrá enterado ¿sí se ha enterado?/*I don't know if you've gotten it? Have you gotten it?*
22 P: sí, sí yo entiendo. *[Yes, yes I understand.]*

We can see that the situation creates a sense of fatigue or lack of trust in spite of the fact that the doctor refers to the patient in a colloquial way, uses small talk, tries to use repetition and questions to confirm things and used the informal you ("tú") and I ("yo"). Still, it is not a fluid conversation.

These examples confirm that there is a lack of linguistic competence, though it could also be interpreted as a lack of collaboration, and we should recognize how this must influence the orientation of these interpersonal relationships.

7.5. Conclusions

The analysis of medical appointments with two different types of speakers, is that, 1. Health care professional – Spanish patient and 2. Health care professional – non-native speaker patient (NNSP) who communicates in Spanish, has made certain features clear. These are:

1. A greater tendency to follow the standard appointment structure and to add sections on bureaucratic procedures and small talk, though this occurs more intensely in Type 2 along with other specificities that we will continue to summarize.
   Specific variants in conversational turn-taking, although they are different depending on type. Given that in Type 1 it is the patient who speaks most while in Type 2 it is typically the doctor who speaks for longer periods of time (when it is really the patient who should speak). Meanwhile, the patient is limited to merely agreeing or disagreeing.
2. A certain propensity to make the medical interview more colloquial using resources such as combining usted + proper name, the use of diminutives, small talk and repetitions.
3. The frequent use of diminutives and other elements of small talk, repetitions and polite conversation (in both cases), though the use of diminutives by Latin-American patients in Type 2 encounters stands out compared to other foreign patients.
4. Variants in the way a person is addressed. Thus, in the doctor's case, the age of the patient seems to be the factor which prompts the doctor to use either the informal you "tú" or the formal you, "usted". When "usted" is used, the doctor tends to soften the tone by adding the patient's name afterwards. In the case of the patient, the use of "usted" tends to prevail in Type 1 while in Type 2, there is certain ambiguity between the use of the informal and formal you, "tú" and "usted" repectively. The informal you, "tú", is sometimes used in contexts where it would not be used by the native speaker. This indicates that more than a lack of pragmatic competence, there is a linguistic lack of competence, but it also shows the influence this can have on the orientation with respect to how the speakers treat one other.
5. Tendency on part of the doctor to "democratize" the intervention more in group 2, while in the case of group 1, both the doctor and native patient tend to continue using "usted", thus keeping with the respect and superiority with which doctors were traditionally viewed in the Spain (not so long ago). We should also mention certain preferences that the doctors have towards the use of "nosotros"/we when a decision needs to be made (eg. diagnosis, treatment). By using "we" the doctor feels like a member of an institution and in this manner, seeks the support of said institution. This said, using "we" also helps to doctor seem less imposing than when "I" is used. Thus, "I" is used in very precise moments with

the intention of establishing his/her presence, especially in the case of Group 2.

In general, these strategies as a whole help create a more relaxed and comfortable environment between doctor and patient. They lend a more positive orientation to the interview with respect to the rapport management with the two types of speakers and thus, help to create a climate of greater trust.

With respect to the foreign patients, certain differences are observed depending on their command of the language. However, we should not pass over the fact that these patients do recognize and use certain social conventions and that they do have a certain command of institutional speech regardless of their origin (Romanian, Bulgarian, Moroccan, Ecuadorian). This can play a role when the time comes to attribute one of the two functions of small talk (phatic or informative function) to what is said; it could be just small talk or it could be part of the patient assessment (asking about country of origin, about family, greetings which require a longer response or personal information). Finally, we should discuss certain differences between those groups where Spanish is the native language and those that speak a language other than Spanish. In the first case, we see the transfer of certain Latin-American Spanish resources to peninsular Spanish, resulting in certain interferences (greater use of diminutives, unusual small talk, different use of the informal you or usted or requesting additional services). This is something which does not occur with the speakers of other languages, though these elements do not negatively affect the mode or orientation by which the relationships between the speakers are established. This definite confirmation of the variations in the structure of the medical appointment based on the type of speaker involved means that further research necessary. We trust that these conclusions will lead to more in-depth research.

All in all, the study shows that there are variations in the strategies implemented when managing interpersonal relationships, although the goal seems to be the same: the desire to positively manage interpersonal relationships during intercultural encounters.

The research presented here is undoubtedly incomplete and requires deeper study. Nonetheless, it is possible to venture some hypotheses or ideas for future studies, such as: the possible influence that linguistic competence bears on the orientation of relationships, the use of different strategies from different speakers depending on their culture or the level of colloquial language used in doctor's speech in different types of medical interviews. I hope that these ideas will be just as interesting to future researchers.

Notes

* A preliminary version of this chapter was published in Spanish in *Pragmática y comunicación intercultural en el mundo hispanohablante, María Elena Placencia & Carmen García (eds.)* Amsterdam/New York, NY : Routledge , 2012. XIX, Foro Hispánico 44, pp. 67-90 with the title "Deme algo, doctor. Estrategias de gestión interrelacional en consultas médicas interculturales".

Practice

This section contains activities to reinforce the information provided in the previous section. The activities can be grouped into two main types: activities for reflection and assimilation of content and activities directed towards research, implementation of skills and strategies in multilingual settings. These activities can be undertaken individually, in pairs or small groups and / or with people from different cultural backgrounds to provide fertile grounds for discussion in class or via email. This will depend largely on the way the book is used (e.g. for self-study, as a textbook, or as support material for any course connected with intercultural communication).

Activity 1.

Summarize the structure of the medical interview. What variations have you seen from the healthcare providers based on the type of patient involved.

Activity 2.

After reading the chapter, provide a definition or explanation of rapport management strategies.

Activity 3.

Pay attention to changes in conversational turn-taking for both types of patients (Type 1: Patients who share the same language as doctors and Type 2: NNSP who do not share the language) and write a brief commentary on the differences (if there are any) in terms of time, amount, information given, etc.

Activity 4.

Look for personal everyday examples of rapport management

Activity 5.

Look up 3-4 bibliographic references on the tendency to democratize the medical consultation and prepare a brief summary of what you find.

Bibliographical references and further reading

Borrell, F. (2004). *Entrevista Clínica. Manual de Estrategias Prácticas.* Barcelona: SEMFYC.

Fairclough, N. (1995). *Critical Discourse Analysis.* London: Longman.

Galanti, G.A. (2004). *Caring for Patients from Different Cultures.* Philadelphia, PA: University of Pennsylvania Press.

Grupo CRIT (2003). *Claves para la Comunicación Intercultural.* Castellón: Universitat Jaume I.

—. (2006). *Culturas Cara a Cara. Relatos y Actividades para la Comunicación Intercultural.* Madrid: Edinumen.

Placencia, M.E and García, C. (2008). "Formas, usos y funciones del *habla de contacto* en español." Sección temática, *Oralia* 11.

Raga Gimeno, F. (2008). *Mediaciones Interculturales.* Valencia: Universitat de València, Lynx.

Spencer-Oatey, H. (2008) (Ed.). "Introduction". In Spencer-Oatey. H. (Ed.) *Culturally Speaking: Culture, Communication and Politeness Theory* (2nd ed.) London: Continuum, 1-8.

Spencer-Oatey, H. and Franklin, P. (2009). *Intercultural Interaction. A Multidisciplinary Approach to Intercultural Communication.* Basingstoke: Palgrave/Macmillan.

Valero-Garcés, C. and Taibi, M. (2004). "Análisis de la interacción comunicativa en contextos institucionales entre proveedores de servicios, usuarios e intermediarios lingüísticos". *Oralia*, 7, 207-228.

Valero-Garcés, C. (2002). "Modificaciones en la conversación institucional. Análisis de los turnos de habla en la entrevista clínica con pacientes inmigrantes". In Luque, G., Bueno, A. and Gabriel T. (Eds.) *Las Lenguas en un Mundo Global.* Jaén: Servicio de Publicaciones de la Universidad, 29-38.

—. (2007). "Doctor-Patient consultations in dyadic and triadic exchanges". In Pöchhacker, F. and Shlesinger, M. (Eds.) *Healthcare Interpreting. Discourse and Interaction.* Amsterdam: John Benjamins, 35-52.

—. (2008). "La conversación de contacto en contextos institucionales: la consulta médica". *Oralia*, 11, 107-131.

CHAPTER EIGHT

HEALTHCARE PROVIDERS AND INTERPRETERS WORKING AS A PROFESSIONAL TEAM

Key Points

- Multidisciplinary efforts and team work in healthcare settings
- Achieving effective communication
- The controversy of the interpreter roles
- Key points in good practice and codes of conduct
- Recommendation to work with interpreters and translators

Key Readings

Bancroft, M. A. et al (2011). "Culture and Mediation". In *The Community Interpreter. A Comprehensive Training Manual*. Columbia, MA: Culture and Language Press, 163-226.

Kelly, N. (2008). "Ethics and Standards". In *Telephone Interpreting: A Comprehensive Guide to the Profession*. Victoria, CA: Trafford Publishing: 93-181.

Hale, S. (2007). "Interdisciplinarity: Community interpreting in the medical context". In *Community Interpreting*. Basingstoke, Hampshire: Palgrave Macmillan: 34-62.

Roat, C. (2003). "How to choose and use a language agency: A guide for health and social service providers who wish to contract with language agencies". California Endowment.

8.1. Introduction

A closer look at healthcare service in many Western countries reveals important changes in the structure of a doctor's visit and in the attitude of medical professionals. As stated in previous chapters, one of the main causes of this is the arrival of migrant populations that bring different languages and cultures and that do not have a good command of the contact language – Spanish in this case. They are new patients with new needs who require new solutions. Multidisciplinary efforts and team work could provide some solutions, given the disparity of opinions and the lack of knowledge people have of one another. This is true not only among professionals and migrants, but also within the professions themselves that, in one form or another, assist migrant populations, that is, doctors, nurses, psychologists, social workers, anthropologists, sociologists, educators, foreign language teachers, linguists, translators and interpreters, professionals in administration, teachers and researchers.

Healthcare providers as well as other professionals should be aware of the extent of the communication difficulties interpreters experience day by day. They should also consider the resources and materials (available or needed) that can also help as a bridge between doctors and patients, and the risks of using bilinguals as ad-hoc interpreters. Among the measures to fill this gap, are the development of materials to offer awareness, the organization of seminars for healthcare providers to show how to work with interpreters and translators, or the introduction of new tools for communicating with foreign patients who do not master the contact language (remote interpreting, specific software, etc.) would minimize serious miscommunication in the mediated medical encounters.

8.2. Bilingual practitioners

A solution often taken is the use of bilingual practitioners. The term "bilingual" is used here simply because it is a commonly used term to denote those who have a working command of two languages, although the term can indicate varying degrees of functionality between the two languages with the fully balanced bilingual being the exception rather than the rule (Baker 2000: 82).

Box 8.1.

Bilingual Person.

An individual who has some degree of proficiency in two languages. A high level of bilingualism is the minimum qualification for a competent interpreter but by itself does not ensure the ability to interpret.

National Standards Guide for Community Interpreting Services. HIN, Canada.

Suitable qualified employees with bilingual language skills can operate in a range of functions and at a range of levels. At a basic level they could work as receptionist welcoming to other – language speakers, take and make telephone calls involving routine message or, at a more specialized level, bilingual practitioners may include trained medical staff.

Box 8.2.

Indeed, bilingual practitioners are particularly useful at higher professional levels in circumstances where working through an interpreter is impractical or challenging. It would not be impossible to work through an interpreter in such cases, and many interpreters do so on a daily basis with some sensitivity, but it might be easier and more effective not to have to. (Corsellis, A. *Public Service Interpreting. First Steps.* Basingstoke, Hampshire: Palgrave Macmillan 2008: 103)

Research and experience demonstrate that bilingual providers of public services need to be supervised, monitored and supported in relation to both their language and professional skills and that duality has to be accommodated in their continuous professional development. It is unfortunate that too often, for reasons of expediency, people are assumed to have sufficient command of a language to do their task properly in a second language when they do not.

Such people may also be exploited and left to cope with matters beyond their professional competence, simply on the basis of what language skills they may possess, without support, recognition or reward and perhaps on top of a normal workload. Just because a doctor or a nurse has a Moroccan or a English mother, it does not necessarily mean that they possess a command of those languages which includes the terminology of their work place or an adequate understanding of the contemporary culture. Nor should they be put in a position where they feel obliged to help out if they do not wish to, or feel under-equipped for the task.

It would be better by far to recognize overtly what languages skills exist and to train bilingual service providers at all levels. In particular, there are contexts in which working through an interpreter without any specific training might be impractical – such as in diagnostic psychiatry and speech therapy- but not impossible. Here the clinical signs and symptoms are embedded in what and how patients communicate. Unless interpreters are medically qualified, it is difficult for them to recognize the implications of what is said and how it is encoded. Nor could a psychiatrist or speech therapist of a different culture find it easy to make sense of what was transferred and treat the patient appropriately.

The bilingual practitioner clearly needs two sets of proven skills: language skills to communicate with their professional colleagues and other-language speaking clients, and the professional or vocational skills to deliver their expertise safely and effectively in the two cultures. Both need to be at the level, and of the type, necessary for the task in hand (Corsellis 2008: 103).

Box 8.3.

Interpreters, translators and bilingual practitioners have different, defined roles but share much in common. In a working world where they are often relatively isolated, they are in a position to give each their mutual professional support over such matters as terminology and procedures.

There may be a number of occasions when people with all three skills sets are working on the same matter. Their combined professional expertise, where appropriate, could bring added value to their tasks. They can certainly add to each other's continuing professional development sessions where, for example, a bilingual lawyer can discuss changes in legislation or legal procedures and then discuss the linguistic implications with interpreter and translator colleagues. (Corsellis, A. *Public Service Interpreting. First Steps.* Basingstoke, Hampshire: Palgrave Macmillan 2008: 117)

The Association of American Medical Colleges (AAMC), whose mission we read is: "The AAMC serves and leads the academic medicine community to improve the health of all," claiming that they are "the only association that brings together education, clinical care, and research to transform health care", also shows its concerns about the use of bilinguals and it offers some recommendations in *Guidelines for Use of Medical Services*:

Box 8.4.

Additional considerations if using the services of an *ad hoc* interpreter (family, friend, employee):

- Respect the patient's desire to use an interpreter of his/her own choosing and document the request
- Use of a minor (under age 18) as an interpreter is only acceptable in emergency situations.

- The use of a family member to interpret for a person with LEP (Limited English Proficiency) cannot be required.
- Family members routinely edit, add, or change the message, and they may try to control the interaction between the patient and the provider instead of facilitating it.
- Talk with the family member/friend/employee to assess his/her language ability and give very clear instructions on how the interaction should progress.
- The fact that an employee is bilingual does not guarantee that the person has the capability to interpret medical language at the level needed.
- Take care not to overburden an employee with interpreting responsibilities if it is not part of his/her job.

Consider issues of conflict of interest/privacy if the *ad hoc* interpreter and patient know each other:
- E.g., in situations where you suspect domestic violence/child abuse and a family member may be the perpetrator.
- E.g., when discussing sensitive issues associated with new diagnoses, STDs, drug use, end of life care, etc.

8.3. Key elements in a profession: the interpreter's roles

Healthcare Interpreting can be defined as the interpreting that takes place in a healthcare setting, in which the interpreter is asked to interpret either consecutively or simultaneously for an individual who does not share the language in which the healthcare service takes place.

Nowadays healthcare providers, as professionals of public services, can no longer expect to work solely with people with whom they share a common language and culture, if they ever did. In order for communication to be effective, however, all parties—service providers as well as users—must be involved in the process. In this regard, we must acknowledge that the situation is also changing for public service employees, who must interact with people who speak other languages and come from different cultures. The process towards adapting to such change will clearly work in combination with a wide range of variables.

Among these variables, there is the health care provider's ability:

- to ask appropriate questions in the most effective way;
- to listen attentively and emphatically to all a patient has to say;
- to understand indirect clues that may lead to further understanding of the patients' problem; and

- to build up a positive and collaborative relationships with the patient.

When a third interlocutor - say an interpreter - is needed, this is required to interpret the healthcare provider's questions and the patient's answers. So the interpreter needs to understand the significance of the information given by both parties, not only in providing direct information in response to questions, but also in providing clues for the health care provider, going beyond words and the literal message. As seen in previous chapters, these intermediaries are often expected to perform a wider role in which the activities of interpreting and mediating are blended, without clear borderlines, in the sense that they do not see the need to translate everything and may omit or add information.

This dimension of the interpreters' role is called mediation. Mediation is often necessary in encounters with foreign population (healthcare centers, schools, police stations, etc.) when the client or provider may not understand what is said, even if the message is expressed accurately and competently. This leads us to the topic of the interpreter roles:

Box 8.5.

Should interpreters only or also mediate? If interpreters mediate, what should they be allowed to do?

Different countries have different answers to these questions and different roles for the interpreters. In some countries, interpreters may not engage in cultural mediation or advocacy while in other countries they are allowed to function as 'active' interpreters.

Beltran Avery (2001: 4) clearly distinguishes these two roles:

Box 8.6.

The "neutral" interpreter

According to the interpreter perspective, the sole function of the medical interpreter is "message passing." The interpreter's only responsibility in the encounter is to provide accurate and complete transmissions of messages conveyed in one language into another language, allowing the patient and provider to interact, as nearly as possible, as if they are engaged in a same language exchange. From this perspective, the interpreter is not an active player in the social encounter occurring between patient and provider. The ideal interpreter presence is unobtrusive and non-relational. There is no recognition that the interpreter could already have connections with the patient community or with the medical institution in which the encounter was occurring. Establishing a relationship with the patient is discouraged.

Neutral interpreters do not initiate any interventions of their own accord and maintain a disengaged presence. The interpreter is there simply as an "instrument," that is, a "black box" in which messages entered in one language and come out in another.

Discussions about the interpreters' roles essentially center on a continuum between interpreting and various forms of mediation. In many circles a tension has long existed between those who believe an interpreter should intervene as needed to "help out" when misunderstandings arise, and those who identified the interpreter as a historically traditional neutral role.

Box 8.7.

The "active" interpreter
In contrast is the active interpreter perspective, in which the interpreter is someone who is likely to hold a variety of responsibilities, beyond that of "message passing." This perspective is championed by interpreters who come from small, closely-knit cultural communities and by those who interpret for communities in which relational ties form the foundation of trust and credibility. The fact that they are bilingual and can negotiate both cultures — theirs and the mainstream culture — often casts them into a position of assuming many other tasks and functions that their community needs to survive.

As Beltran Avery continues writing, this perspective incorporates the likelihood that the interpreter often is a part of or has knowledge of the patient's cultural context that the provider might not and knowledge of the culture of medicine that the patient might not. It recognizes that such knowledge is central to the ability to understand the "intended meaning" of the messages that are being conveyed and make the appropriate equivalent conversions. Because of this the interpreter is sometimes required to assume an active role in the clinical encounter. For example, if a cultural factor such as a belief, assumption, or value, is creating a misunderstanding that affects the goals of the encounter, the interpreter would be expected to intervene. In such situations, the interpreter has the legitimate option of alerting both parties to the miscommunication, offering suggestions as to what could be impeding mutual understanding, and assisting both parties to explore and negotiate these impediments to understanding.

Between these two roles – the neutral and the active - there is some distance and intermediary roles identified by The *National Council on Interpreting in Health Care* (NCIHC) in the USA as:

1. Conduit: Literal interpretation in the first person without omissions, editing, polishing, or outside conversations.
2. Clarifier: clarify linguistic misunderstandings
3. Cultural broker: address cultural barriers
4. Advocate: address systematic barriers. Take action on behalf of a patient that does not deal with the message that one person is trying to pass on to the other.

The incremental intervention model, or "pyramid" model (Roat 2006) includes the four roles:

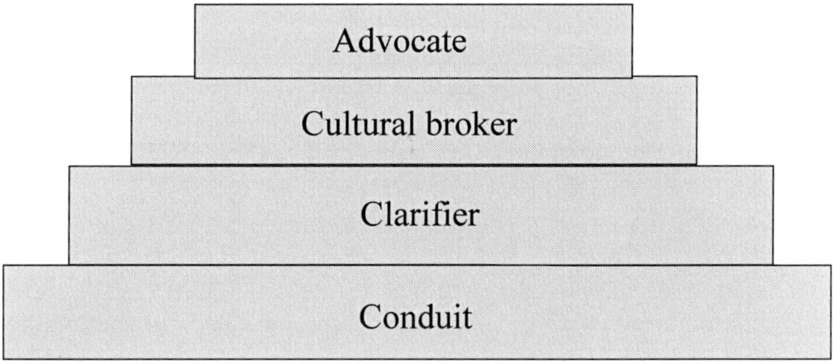

Figure 8.1: The incremental intervention model

Box 8.8.

The model of the incremental intervention
In this model, the role of the interpreter is seen as flexible, ranging from the least intrusive role of conduit, to clarifier, to culture broker and finally, to the most intrusive role of advocate. The model recognizes the need for the interpreter to stay in the background and to support communication and relationship-building directly between patient and provider, while at the same time allowing the interpreter a legitimate way to intervene if she perceives that a misunderstanding is occurring. The level of intrusion that is least invasive yet will adequately facilitate understanding between

patient and provider dictates the choice of role. Movement across the boundaries of different roles is determined by the demands of the situation. (Beltran Avery, B. *The Role of the Health Care Interpreter. An Evolving Dialogue.* 2001:15)

8.4. Techniques and modes of Interpreting

Attention could also be paid to the different strategies and techniques or modes interpreters use depending on the circumstances:

The two main modes of interpreting are simultaneous and consecutive interpreting.

Simultaneous interpreting: the interpreter will be listening, changing the language, and speaking all at once. It saves time and gives immediacy and flow to the conversation. It is often used in court and can be very useful in medical situations as well.

Box 8.9.

"You can help a lot by speaking at a leisurely normal pace, being extra careful about your diction, and speaking very slightly louder than usual because the interpreter can hear her own voice as well" (Cambridge 2013).

Consecutive Interpreting. There are two forms of consecutive interpreting:

1. Long or classic consecutive is usually used in conference interpreting settings, where the interpreter listens to the totality of the speaker's comments or a significant passage and then reconstitutes the speech with the help of notes taken while listening.
2. Sequential or short consecutive interpreting is used in court interpreting as well as most forms of community interpreting and operates at the sentence level instead of working with paragraphs or entire speeches.

In this form of interpreting, the interpreter may interrupt the speaker and ask him/her to repeat, clarify or rephrase so as to ensure accuracy and completeness in the delivery of the message.

Box 8.10.

Consecutive interpreting: the interpreter listens and takes notes while one person speaks, and then relays the message. Taking notes is a sign of competence. When the message contains a lot of hard facts such as dates and times, names and places, there is less risk of forgetting something vital if it has been written down. Cambridge's recommendation for speakers is: "Always finish the thought before you stop speaking to allow interpretation".

Some other techniques follow:

Relay Interpreting. An interpreting process in which two individuals attempting a conversation communicate through two interpreters, each of whom speaks only one of the two languages required as well as a common third language. This type of interpreting is also called double relay. It should be avoided whenever possible because it increases the risk of inaccuracies in interpreting.

Remote Interpreting. Interpreting provided by an interpreter who is not in the presence of the speakers, e.g., interpreting via telephone or videoconferencing

Sight Translation. Conversion from written material in one language to a spoken version in another language. It also occurs when an instant oral version is required of a written text.

Signed Language. Visual-spatial languages used by Deaf people. Signed Languages are natural languages with their own grammatical structures and lexicon. Some organizations: American Sign Language (ASL), European Forum of Sign Language Interpreters (EFSIL) Federación Española de Interpretes de Lengua de Signos (FILSE).

Whispered Simultaneous Interpreting. Interpreting that takes place whereby the interpreter is seated next to one or more LEP/LFP persons and whispers in the target language the content of the speech. Also called "chuchotage"

Video Conference Interpreting. Remote interpreting that makes use of a video camera when one or more of the interpreting parties are not present at the same location. It enables the parties to see and hear each other via a television monitor.

(National Standards Guide for Community Interpreting Services. HIN.Canada)

8.5. Telephone Interpreting

Telephone interpreting deserves special attention; its use in remote interpreting increases every day. Just a paragraph from the article *Medical Interpreter's Guide to Telephone Interpreting* by Nataly Kelly (2008) will help to understand its use and interest.

Telephone interpreting saw an increase in use in areas where in-person interpreters were not historically easy to access. Those in need of the service were given the telephonic option first and foremost. The use of telephone interpreting continues to rapidly expanded to many other areas where an interpreter service is not available.

As Kelly points out, providers who favor telephone interpreting often feel that they are able to develop a therapeutic rapport with the patient that is not triadic in nature, but seems more dualistic as the interpreter is truly invisible (not physically present). There are also many situations that are not well-suited to telephone interpreting such as giving bad news, long interactions, procedures that require demonstrations, settings that prevent the patient from being close to a telephone, and situations where visual cues may be especially important, such as patient education and teaching scenarios.

However, for some languages, especially in emergency settings, telephone interpreting may be the only option available, even in a less than ideal situation. The recommendation is that, whenever telephone interpreting is used in those types of settings, the provider needs to be sure to describe the procedures and setting with as much detail as possible to help the interpreter maintain the necessary level of quality. Likewise, telephone interpreters in these settings must request clarification frequently to ensure accuracy of comprehension prior to interpreting.

Box 8.11.

In what settings is telephone interpreting preferable to onsite interpreting, and vice versa?:

There are many situations for which telephone interpreting is the most appropriate modality. For example, when a provider has to call his/her patient, telephone interpreting is really the best option. When a triage nurse has to ascertain the patient's condition quickly, telephone interpreting might be the quickest option, and therefore, the best option to ensure the safety of the patient. Front desk queries, registration processes, and other communications of this nature that do not involve a provider frequently lend themselves to telephone interpreting.

There are also many situations that are not well-suited to telephone interpreting, such as giving bad news, long interactions, procedures that require demonstrations, settings that prevent the patient from being close to a telephone, and situations where visual cues may be especially important, such as patient education and teaching scenarios.

However, for some languages, especially in emergency settings, telephone interpreting may be the only option available, even in less than ideal situations. Whenever telephone interpreting is used in those types of settings, the provider needs to be sure to describe the procedures and setting with as much detail as possible to help the interpreter maintain the necessary level of quality. Likewise, telephone interpreters in these settings must request clarification frequently to ensure accuracy of comprehension prior to interpreting.

Kelly, N. (2008). *Telephone Interpreting: A Comprehensive Guide to the Profession.*

8.6. Code of conduct and guide of good practice

A professional interpreter, as any professional, must follow a code of ethics.

Box 8.12.

The four basic principles of any code of conduct in the interpreting profession are:

Confidentiality: Respect others' rights to privacy.

Impartiality: Do not take sides with either party.

Accuracy: Make sure the message is accurate and appropriate in the new cultural context.

Integrity: Be honest with yourself and your abilities or skills when accepting a translation/interpreting job.

These principles take on very different names and purposes in the different codes of conduct and good practice guidelines that have been developed and published by institutions or centres that are directly related to PSIT. Often they are very basic principles or recommendations that people who work as interpreters or translators in these centres must observe. The websites hosted by professional associations, as the ones that follow, are excellent resources for interpreters. They provide much useful information as well as links to other relevant websites.

AUSIT (*Australian Institute of Interpreters and Translators Incorporated*)
CCHCP (Cross Cultural Health Care Program)
CHIA (*California Healthcare Interpreters Association*)
IMIA (*International Medical Interpreters Association*)
IoL (*Institute of Linguists, United Kingdom*)
MMIA (Massachusetts Medical Interpreters Association)
NAATI (National Accreditation Authority for Translators and Interpreters, Australia)
NCIHC (*National Council of Interpreting in Health Care, USA*)
NRPSI (National Register of Public Service Interpreters, UK)
RID (Registry of Interpreters for the Deaf, EE UU and Canada)

8.7. Is an interpreter necessary? Working with an interpreter

Increasingly, Codes of Conduct or Guides of Good Practice tend to include recommendations for the service providers about to work with interpreters and translators. Some examples follow amongst many others.

Box 8.13.

Is an interpreter necessary?

"The client speaks English well enough when they want."

Going to court or hospital is not "when they want" and they may be afraid or in pain. The kind of English they will hear there can be difficult enough to understand even for people who have spoken English all their lives. As a professional in your own field, you naturally want provide the highest standards of safe, effective service. This means good communication, so the interpreter is for your benefit as much as the client's. There have been infamous examples of harm being done by lack of an interpreter, or poor interpretation. Research has shown that communications are improved when a professional, trained and registered interpreter is called to assist in communicating across language and culture. Iqbal Begum (R. v Iqbal Begum (1991) 93 Criminal appeal Reports 96), and Victoria Climbié (see the Laming Report, 2003) are two examples. Cambridge, J. (2013). *Working effectively through a professional interpreter*.

Following the recommendations by the Association of American Medical Colleges (AAMC) in their *Guidelines for Use of Medical Interpreter Services* some useful steps are:

Box 8.14.

Assessing the Need for a Medical Interpreter

A patient with limited contact language proficiency (individuals, who, because the contact language is not their primary language, have a limited ability to speak, read, write, or understand the contact language) presents and requires a medical interpreter:

A. Call your hospital's trained medical interpreter:

- First, brief the medical interpreter about the goals of this patient contact.
- Request the medical interpreter to interpret in a conduit fashion.
- Ask the medical interpreter to clarify in her/his own words whenever a misunderstanding due to cultural differences might occur.
- For written instructions, always use a translator[1], if available.

Otherwise, ask the medical interpreter to translate (in writing) basic instructions for the patient.

B. If the patient is alone and no medical interpreter is available, use a telephonic interpreter and refer to instructions in part A.

C. Always document, in detail, the use of the medical interpreter or translator in the patient's chart.

If a trained medical interpreter is not available:

D. If use of an *ad hoc* interpreter is necessary (family, friend, or employee):

- First, assess the interpreter's level of contact language proficiency and its sufficiency for the type of interaction expected.
- Instruct the interpreter to interpret exactly what the patient says and not to edit or summarize any information.
- Never use a minor (under age 18) to interpret personal information unless in an emergency situation.
- Always be aware of potential issues of confidentiality or conflicts of interest between the patient and the ad hoc interpreter.
- Ask the *ad hoc* interpreter if he/she is comfortable with the situation in which he/she will serve as an interpreter.

8.8. Working with a Medical Interpreter

The *International Medical Interpreters Association* (IMIA), in the *IMIA Guide on Working with Medical Interpreters,* after providing a definition of a medical interpreter as "a trained professional bound by a code of ethics", mentione the three steps in an interpreting even followed by a set of recommendations for the service providers as seen in Box 8.15:

Box 8.15.

Pre-Session

- A good cultural and linguistic match between patient and interpreter can avoid many potential problems. If possible, when requesting an interpreter consider: (social/ethnic issues, dialects)

- Learn how the patient prefers to be called

- Discuss eye contact, seating/positioning

- Establish a rapport with the interpreter

- Explain the purpose of the session

- Encourage the interpreter to ask clarifying questions (clarifier role) for accuracy

- Ask the interpreter to explain the nature of any independent conversation with the client or you to the other party during the session to promote transparency and impartiality of all parties

- Make sure you have forms in the client's care language and or go over the non-translated form with the interpreter carefully before the interview

During Session

- Allow interpreters to introduce themselves and "screen" client's speech

- Allow the interpreter to best position themselves to promote direct eye contact between provider/patient wherever possible

- Do not make comments to the interpreter that you don't mean to be interpreted to the patient

- Let the interpreter explain the ground rules for communicating with an interpreter:

- Everything said by both parties will be interpreted

- Speak in short phrases so the interpreter will be able to interpret more easily

- Tell the patient that what they say is confidential; will not reveal anything about the interview

- Ask the patient if they have any questions about the interpreting process

- Talk to your client by talking to them in the first person and not in the third person as in 'Tell him xyz"

- Be patient, and encourage the interpreter's understanding

- Respect the interpreter's judgment, if the interpreter insists that a questions is inappropriate, discuss it after the session

- Use time efficiently

- Use simple language and avoid jargon, technical terms, and slang, it is the provider's responsibility to ensure that the patient is understanding via teach back and other methods

- Speak in a normal tone and speed. Speak in the first and second persons only (not third person). Correct: "*What medications are you taking?*"

- Incorrect: "Please ask him what medications he is taking?"

Post-Session

- Discuss issues that could not be adequately discussed during the session

- Thank the interpreter

Some basic guidelines also to be considered are:

- Interpretation should be in a consecutive mode.
- Position yourself so that you face the patient rather than the interpreter.
- Talk with the patient in the first person (using "I").
- Maintain direct eye contact with the patient.
- Do not direct your questions or inquiries to the interpreter
- Ask the patient to repeat any instructions and explanations given to insure that they are understood.

8.9. Clients and service providers' responsibilities

Clients and service providers as members of the team that makes efficient communication possible when working with interpreters are also key elements in the process of communication. They also share some responsibilities. The chats below (Boses 8.16, 8.17) contain some of the recommendation in the *National Standard Guide for Community Interpreting Services* (Canada):

8.9.1. Responsibilities of Clients

Box 8.16.

The client shall:

1. Always inform the Interpreting Service Provider (agency or interpreter) of any known risks and provide any advice, protection and safety measures generally available to participants in the interpreted event. The interpreter shall never be forced to enter a situation that poses a risk to his/her health and well being.
2. Respect the Standards of Practice and Ethical Principles at all times.
3. Provide as much information as possible about the requested assignment such as background and parallel texts and speaker's notes. The information will assist the interpreter in researching the subject and familiarizing him/herself with the subject.

Any related documentation, previously translated files or glossaries related to the case are essential to the successful completion of the assignment.

When working with interpreters, the Client should:

1. Book additional time beyond that required in a non-interpreted encounter.
2. Avoid long, complex sentences, the use of slang, idiomatic expressions, highly technical vocabulary or jargon.
3. Speak clearly and at a moderate pace.
4. Talk directly to the LEP/LFP party, not to the interpreter.
5. Never ask the interpreter for his/her opinion.
6. For long assignments, provide breaks at appropriate intervals since accuracy declines with time.
7. Pause frequently to allow the interpreter to render all the information.
8. Be aware of non-verbal communication.
9. Encourage the interpreter to request clarification as required.

10. Provide an adequate working environment.

11. Always attempt to ensure the proper mode of interpreting is used (consecutive or simultaneous).

8.9.2. Responsibilities of Interpreting Service Providers - ISP

Box 8.17.

Organizations that contract community interpreters should have documented procedures in place for selecting people in accordance with the National Standard Guide for Community Interpreting Services. Organizations must ensure that the competencies required are maintained and updated.

Interpreting Service Providers coordinate the provision of interpretation services with clients and interpreters.

Responsibilities to the Client

The Interpreting Service Provider shall:

1. Ensure all interpreters hired or contracted are qualified professionals capable of performing the specified task.

2. Disclose the interpreter's qualifications to the client especially if the interpreter available does not meet the requirements for the specific setting.

3. Brief the client on how to work effectively with interpreters.

4. Inform the client promptly if an interpreter is not available in the requested language.

5. Provide the client with a detailed Client-ISP agreement specifying pricing, terms, policies and procedures for interpreting assignments.

Responsibilities to the Interpreter

The Interpreting Service Provider shall:

1. Provide the interpreter with detailed information about the assignment. This includes:

a. Requesting context/materials/documentation from the client, as applicable.

b. Providing any glossaries or resources available.

c. Providing administrative details such as complete address, contact information, etc.

2. Ensure proper working conditions for the interpreter. This includes:

a. Promoting an adequate working environment.

b. Briefing the client about the interpreter's needs.

c. Providing the required number of interpreters or team of interpreters if applicable.

3. Pay within a reasonable timeframe and/or according to established agreement between the parties.
4. Clearly establish and document terms and conditions of the working relationship with interpreters.
(National Standards Guide for Community Interpreting Services. HIN, Canada)

8.10. Working with a translator

This distinction between interpreter and translator, and translation and interpreting is fundamental and not always taken into account.

Box 8.18.

Translation. The process of transposing the meaning of a written text from one language (source) to the other (target) by producing an equivalent target text that retains the elements of meaning, form and tone.
Translator. Person who renders the meaning of a written text in a source language to a target language by producing an equivalent written target text that retains the elements of meaning, form and tone.
(*National Standards Guide for Community Interpreting, Canada*)

The skills to work with a translator are similar in many ways and, and following Corsellis (2003), include the skills and understanding to:

- Recognize when a translation is needed. There can be few patients, for example, who can remember exactly what the pharmacist or doctor said to them later –especially in the middle of the night with a crying baby. A short translation of the prescription, which includes: the name of the medication, how much is to be taken, when and how, the possible side effects and what to do about them if they occur could save a life.
- Identify the language correctly (an obvious point which also clearly applies to choosing an interpreter).
- Take appropriate action where the language in question has no written form or whether the intended reader has difficulties in literacy.
- Assess the text to be translated e.g. its complexity, technical detail – and its purpose. The last differs in the public service context between, for example, a formal legal document and a set of instructions for weaning babies.
- Contact and commission a suitable translator.
- Allow sufficient time for a competent translation to be done.

- Brief the translator and be ready to answer any queries and clarifications necessary.
- Consider with the translator what should be done in such matters as non-functional equivalencies, where a word or term does not exist in the other language, and whether and how any different starting points of the intended reader should be accommodated.
- Clarify deadlines and mode of lay-out and presentation – remembering, for example, that where the second language text is to be read from right to left any photographs and the like in the original will have to be re-positioned.
- Explain and facilitate any security requirements.
- Clarify any cross checking or proof reading arrangements.

Box 8.19.

Translation is a precise art and, unlike the interpreter, the translator cannot see and evaluate the individual reader or assess the readers' response, nor is there often the possibility of providing clarification while the translated text is being read.

Remember, translating is not interpreting. They are different professions and use very different skills.

8.11. Stress in the team. Interpreters are not machines

Working as a public service in general, and healthcare interpreters in particular, require the ability to work in difficult settings and deal with sensitive issues, and consequently work under strong psychological and emotional stress. Interpreters must listen and transfer the messages of people who, in many cases, exhibit violent or nervous behaviour because they have suffered painful experiences throughout their lives.

The staff members can be a source of stress as well. However, even when both the client and service provider behave professionally and courteously, other common stress factors will arise. Clearly, numerous occupational demands – such as mastering linguistic skills or possessing the political, cultural, social and religious knowledge of the public service interpreting client - can affect the overall interpreting task and may contribute to interpreter's stress and burnout. As in the case of many professions, the daily high demand of the job can consume the interpreter's energy.

Nowadays there is an increasing interest in studying stress, and research is usually accompanied by suggestions and recommendations to help professionals to overcome this stress. Training is the most frequently mentioned suggestion; but stress is a widespread and costly problem, and there are very few actions taken and the majority of solutions proposed will never be implemented. The causes of stress are the workload, time pressure and hassle, but how we do handle these problems?

Empirical research has shown that there is a wide range of symptoms of stress including subjective symptoms (fatigue, depression, burn out); behavioural (unfriendliness, sociopathy); cognitive (poor concentration, fear); physical (high cholesterol, heart diseases); and organizational (performance decrements) (Riccardi, Marinuzzi and Zecchin, 2002); and studies related to interpreting have also shown that these symptoms may be present in interpreters and might lead to consequences such as depression (Navarro 2012, Musacchio 2013); burn-out (Watson, 1987, Maslach & Leiter, 1997); or fear (Magalhães, 2012) among others.

The following study by Musacchio (2013) will help to give a more accurate picture of the psychological and emotional impact of stress on interpreters.

Marianna Musacchio (2013), in "The Psychological Impact on Interpreters in the Mental Health Setting: The Case of Ulysses' syndrome" (*El impacto psicológico de los intérpretes en el ámbito de la salud mental: el caso del síndrome de Ulise*s) concentrates on a very specific topic: analyzing stress in the mental health setting. She also wanted to study if migrant patients attending mental health consultations tended to suffer from the Immigrant Syndrome with Chronic and Multiple Stress (Ulysses' Syndrome, Achotegui 2003) and if this condition could affect the interpreter.

She developed three different semi-structured surveys for migrant patients (30 answers *in situ*), doctors (10 answers *in situ*) and interpreters (24 *in situ* and email). The results of the analysis showed that the experiences of these patients are often tragic and the interpreters who are working in these kinds of consultations exhibited a deep emotional involvement, one which they must be able to control in order to avoid suffering indirect trauma.

The results also indicate that migrants appreciate the presence of an interpreter during the consultation, and this does not alter the balance of the communication between the patient and the doctor, contradicting the opinion of some psychiatrists who believe that the presence of a third (unknown) element (the interpreter) could interfere with their work. The conclusion, for interpreters working with sensitive issues (such as mental disorders) can cause stress, but the patients suffering from these disorders exhibit more trust and feel more at ease when there is an interpreter present. As for the interpreters, the results from the survey and interviews indicate that the more specialized the interpreter and the greater his or her knowledge and "closeness" to the Ulysses syndrome, the less he / she was affected by the patients' conditions and stress. This finding calls attention to the need for specialized training.

Likewise, the surveys conducted with health care staff (psychiatrists, psychologists) working with migrant patients show that, in general, these professionals feel a significant need to help them, not just from a linguistic standpoint, but also from a cultural and psychological one. In fact, some doctors tend to exhibit signs of stress, nervousness and irritability due to incomprehension and misunderstandings, problems which can easily be resolved through an interpreter who helps save time, avoids stress and guarantees greater success within the consultation.

However, the study also highlights contradictory points of view among the staff concerning the use of interpreters. This may indicate the lack of awareness of the interpreter's roles on the part of the service provider and the need for training both the medical staff and the interpreters who often work as freelance interpreters with potentially limited experience in this setting.

Among the resources or strategies pointed out by the psychologists in order to cope with this situation are: Writing a report or summary; looking to family members; walk; reflect; work or study; share the experience with colleagues, or participate in leisure activities.

The above example shows that working as medical interpreters may require the ability to work in difficult settings and deal with sensitive issues, and to consequently work under strong psychological and emotional stress as in any other profession.

Box 8.20.

Interpreters are not machines. The intense work of interpreting in healthcare settings is often stressful.

Patients are often frightened, confused, tense or uncertain and may react in negative ways. This may result from frustration at the slow (or quick) pace of the session, difficulty in making themselves understood or in understanding what the provider is saying. Patients may direct their feelings at the provider and sometimes at the interpreter.

Providers, on the other hand, may behave in a frustrated manner, appearing to be hurried or critical of the patient, or even of the interpreter. These interactions may cause interpreters to feel uncomfortable, sometimes inadequate, and even angry.

Interpreters may find themselves suddenly interpreting emotionally-charged subject matter, such as a diagnosis of a terminal illness, a bad prognosis for an illness or injury, or a death announcement. At other times, interpreters may be uncertain about the patient's or provider's expectations, while perceiving tension and frustration in the session. Interpreters may already feel under stress. They may be concerned about making mistakes, working for the first time with a provider or a patient. They could be working with individuals with difficult personalities, calming an agitated or fearful patient, or interpreting complex subject matter and technical terminology. It is critical for interpreters to be aware of their own level of emotional responses to what is happening around them, and to know how to protect their own health and well-being.

(California Healthcare Interpreting Association (CHIA)

8.12. Conclusion

As a conclusion a set of recommendations follows:

- Hospitals should develop explicit policies or plans related to the provision of language services for patients with limited knowledge of the contact language.
- Bilingual clinicians and staff should be assessed for language proficiency if they provide direct services or care to patients with limited English.
- Volunteer interpreters should have their language proficiency assessed and be trained in medical interpreting.
- Hospitals should require that all staff, including clinical staff, receive education on the critical importance of language services to patient care and training on how to access language services.
- All hospitals should know who their patients and work force are and work to meet the language needs of all of their patients.

(adapted from the study "Talking With Patients How Hospitals Use Bilingual Clinicians and Staff to Care for Patients with Language Needs", supported by The California Endowment.)

Practice

This section contains activities to reinforce the information provided in the previous section. The activities can be grouped into two main types: activities for reflection and assimilation of content and activities directed towards research, implementation of skills and strategies in multilingual settings. These activities can be undertaken individually, in pairs or small groups and / or with people from different cultural backgrounds to provide fertile grounds for discussion in class or via email. This will depend largely on the way the book is used (e.g. for self-study, as a textbook, or as support material for any course connected with intercultural communication).

Activity 1.

After reading the paper summarize the functions of a healthcare provider in multilingual settings

Activity 2.

According to the information provided, identify the skills that service providers must have to work with interpreters.

Activity 3.

As discussed in the previous pages, mastering a language is not enough to ensure being a good interpreter and/or translator. Nonetheless, most of the work of transferring information from a language that is practically unknown to migrants or vice versa (from the majority language into the minority one) is normally performed by individuals who more or less know both languages, but who have not received specialized training and who will not have the opportunity to do so, as it does not exist. In order to verify this information, do some research in your area on the language services offered or materials available in other languages and who has translated them. Comment on your findings.

Activity 4.

Read the following quotation and write a comment comparing with your experience or healthcare providers you know:

"Heathcare providers would introduce the case to the interpreter, inform her or him of the goals of the consultation, the nature of the condition, of any procedures and provide any other relevant information. The interpreter, on the other hand, would explain his or her role, maintaining eye contact with the patient, seating arrangements, etc.) and alert the medical practitioner of obvious cultural differences, if any. Ideally the interpreter would receive information on the case before the day of the assignment in order to prepare thoroughly (…). If the interpreter and the health care provider have worked together before, some of the contents of the briefing session would not need to be repeated" (Hale 2007: 61).

Bibliographic references and further reading

Achotegui, J. (2002). "Immigrants living in extreme situation: immigrant Syndrome with chronic and multiple stress (the Ulysses syndrome)". http://www.fhspereclaver.org/migra-salut-mental/Ulises/Ulysses%20text%202%20english-1.pdf [Last accessed April 30th, 2014].

Bancroft, M.A. et al (2011). "Culture and Mediation". *The Community Interpreter. A Comprehensive Training Manual*. Columbia, MA: Culture and Language Press, 163-226.

Beltran Avery, M.P. (2001). "The Role of the Heath Care Interpreter: An Evolving Dialogue". *The National Council on Interpreting in Health Care Working Paper Series.* Washington, DC: NCIHC. [www.ncihc.org [Last accessed April 30th, 2014].

Cambridge, J. (2003). "Unas ideas sobre la interpretación en los centros de salud". In Valero-Garcés, C. (Ed.) *Traducción e Interpretación en los Servicios Públicos. Contextualización, Actualidad y Futuro.* Granada: Comares, 57-59.

—. (2013). "Working Effectively Through a Professional Interpreter". http://publicserviceinterpreting.com/category/public-service-providers/guidance-on-working-effectively-with-interpreters/ [Last accessed April 30th, 2014].

Cost-effectiveness of Language Services Project Literature Review. (2008). http://www.imiaweb.org/uploads/pages/197.pdf [Last accessed April 30th, 2014].

Grubbs, V. et al. (2006). "Effect of Awareness of Language Law on language Access in the Health Care Setting". *Journal of General Internal Medicine*, 21(7), 683–688.

Hale, S. (2007). "Interdisciplinarity: Community Interpreting in the Medical Context". *Community Interpreting*. Hampshire: Palgrave Macmillan: 34-62.

Healthcare Interpretation Network (2009). *National Standards Guide for Community Interpreteng Services*. HIN: Toronto, Canada.

International Medical Interpreters Association (2007). *Medical Interpreting Standards of Practice*. Boston, MA: IMIA.

Kelly, N. (2008). "Ethics and Standards". *Telephone Interpreting: A Comprehensive Guide to the Profession*. Victoria, CA: Trafford Publishing: 93-181.

Ku, L. and Flores, G. (2005). "Pay Now or Pay Later: Providing Interpreter Services in Health Care". *Health Affairs*, 24(2), 435-444.

Magalhães E. (2012). "Afraid? Who is afraid?". *The ATA Chronicles*. http://ewandromagalhaes.tempsite.ws/ARQUIVOS/PDF/ATA_CHRONICLE_MAR12.PDF [Last accessed April 30th, 2014].

Maslach, C., and Leiter, M.P. (1997). *The Truth about Burnout: How Organizations cause Personal Stress and What to do about it*. (2nd ed.). San Francisco, CA: Jossey-Bass.

Musacchio, M. (2013). *El Impacto Psicológico de los Intérpretes en el Ámbito de la Salud Mental: El Caso del síndrome de Ulises*. [Unpublished Master's Thesis]. Universidad de Alcalá, Madrid, Spain.

Navarro Moreno, S. (2012). *Interpretación en los Servicios Públicos. Impacto Psicológico y Emocional en el Intérprete. Análisis de Casos y Situaciones*. [Unpublished Master's Thesis]. Universidad de Alcalá, Madrid, Spain.

Rahman, I. Hirsch, J. and Shah, S. (2007). "Overcoming Language Barriers in the Criminal Justice System: Can Language Assistance TechnologyHelp?" http://www.empirejustice.org/archive/larc/newsitedesign/LEPTopics/LE/PoliceChiefArticle/Police%20Chief%20Magazine%20-%20View%20Article.htm [Last accessed: April 30th, 2014].

Riccardi, A., Marinuzzi, G., Zecchin, S. (2002). "Interpretation and stress". *Interpreting in the 21st Century*. Amsterdam/Philadelphia: John Benjamins, 93-105.

Roat, C. (2003). *How to choose and use a language agency: A guide for health and social service providers who wish to contract with language agencies*. Menlo Park, CA: The California Endowment.

—. (2006). *Certification of Health Care Interpreters in the United States: A Primer, a Status Report and Consideration for National Certification*. Menlo Park, CA: The California Endowment.

Sánchez-Reyes, S. and Martín Casado, M. (2005). "Argumentos a favor de la implantación de un servicio de intérpretes en los hospitales". In Valero-Garcés, C. *Traducción como Mediación entre Lenguas y Culturas. Translation as Mediation or How to Bridge the Cultural Gap*. Alcalá de Henares: Servicio de Publicaciones de la Universidad de Alcalá.

Stone, D. (2007). *30 Days to Taming Your Stress*. Eufene, Oregon: Harvest House Publishers.

Valero-Garcés, C. (2006). "Emotional and Psychological Effects on Interpreters in Public Services. A Critical Factor to Bear in Mind". http://www.translationdirectory.com/article537.htm [Last accessed April 30th, 2014].

Watson, J. (1987). "Interpreter burnout". *Journal of Interpretation*, 4, 79–85.

REFERENCES

Achotegui, J. (2000). "Los duelos de la migración". *Medicina y Cultura.* In Perdiguero, E. and Comelles, J.M. Barcelona: Editorial Bellaterra, 88-100.

—. (2002). *La Depresión en los Inmigrantes: Una Perspectiva Transcultural.* Barcelona: Ediciones Mayo.

—. (2002). "Immigrants living in extreme situation: immigrant syndrome with chronic and multiple stress (the Ulysses syndrome)". http://www.fhspereclaver.org/migra-salut-mental/Ulises/Ulysses%20text%202%20english-1.pdf [Last accessed April 30th, 2014].

Aerny Perreten N., Ramasco Gutiérrez M., Cruz Maceín J., Rodríguez Rieiro C., Garabato González S. and Rodríguez Laso, A. (2010). "La salud y sus determinantes en la población inmigrante de la Comunidad de Madrid". *Gaceta Sanitaria*, 24(2), 136-144.

Ainsworth-Vaughn, N. (1998). *Claiming Power in Doctor-Patient Talk.* New York: Oxford University Press.

Alonso, A. Huerga H and Morera J. (2003). *Guía de Atención al Inmigrante*. SMMFYC. Madrid: Ergon.

Asnani, MR. (2009). "Patient-physician communication". *West Indian Med J*, 58(4), 357-61.

Atkinson, P. (1999). "Medical discourse, evidentiality and the construction of professional responsibility". In Sarangi, S. and Roberts, C. (Eds.) *Talk, Work, and Institutional Order: Discourse in Medical, Mediation and Management Settings*. New York: Mouton de Gruyter, 75-106.

Balaban, C. (2012). *Investigación sobre consentimientos informados. Comparación de la situación entre España y Rumania.* [Unpublished Master's Thesis]. Universidad de Alcalá, Madrid, Spain.

Bancroft, M and Rubio-Fitzpatrick, L. (2011). *The Community Interpreter. A Comprehensive Training Manual.* Columbia, MA: Culture and Language Press.

Beltran Avery, M.P. (2001). "The Role of the Heath Care Interpreter: An Evolving Dialogue". *The National Council on Interpreting in Health Care Working Paper Series*. Washington, DC: NCIHC. [www.ncihc.org [Last accessed April 30th, 2014].

Benavides, F.G., Nolasco, A., Jiménez, L., Gonzáles, C., López, J.M., Pérez, E. et al. (1987). "Aplicación y Validez de un Cuestionario para

Medir la Satisfacción de los Usuarios de un Centro de Salud". *Atención Primaria,* 4(2), 91-95.

Borrell, F. (2004). *Entrevista Clínica. Manual de Estrategias Prácticas*. Barcelona: SEMFYC.

Byrne, J., Napier, A. and Cuschieri, A. (1988). "How informed is signed consent?". *BMJ,* 296, 839-840.

Cambridge, J. (1999). "Information loss in bilingual medical interviews through an untrained interpreters". *The Translator,* 5(2), 201-219.

—. (2002). "Interlocutor roles and the pressures as interpreters". In Valero-Garcés, C. and Mancho, G. (Eds.) *Traducción e Interpretación en los Servicios Públicos: Nuevas Necesidades para Nuevas Realidades/New Needs for New Realities*. Alcalá de Henares: Servicio de Publicaciones de la Universidad, 121-126.

—. (2003). "Unas ideas sobre la interpretación en los centros de salud". In Valero-Garcés, C. (Ed.) *Traducción e Interpretación en los Servicios Públicos. Contextualización, Actualidad y Futuro.* Granada: Comares, 57-59.

—. (2013). "Working Effectively Through a Professional Interpreter." http://publicserviceinterpreting.com/category/public-service-providers/guidance-on-working-effectively-with-interpreters/ [Last accessed April 30th, 2014].

Candlin, C. (2000). "General editor's preface". In Coupland, J. (Ed.) *Small Talk*. London: Longman, 13-20.

Candlin, C. and Candlin, S. (2003). "Health care communication: A problematic site for applied linguistics research". *Annual Review of Applied Linguistics* 23, 134-154.

Carrasco Garrido, P., Jiménez García, R., Hernández Barrera, V., et al. (2009). "Significant differences in the use of healthcare resources of native-born and foreign born in Spain". *BMC Public Health*, 9, 201-213.

Carballo, M. (2006). *El Impacto de la Migración en la Salud: el Caso de la Diabetes*. Centro Internacional para la Migración y la Salud. Encuentro en la Escuela de Verano de Salud Pública.

Case, S. (1988). "Cultural differences not deficiencies: an analysis of managerial women's language". In Rose, S. and Harwood, L. (Eds.) *Women's Careers: Pathways and Pitfalls*. New York: Praeger, 41-63.

Cicourel, A. (1992). "The interpenetration of communicative contexts: Examples from medical encounters". In Goodwin, C. and Duranti, A. (Eds.) *Rethinking Context*. Cambridge: Cambridge University Press, 291-310.

—. (1995). "Medical speech events as resources for inferring differences inexpert-novice diagnostic reasoning". In Quasthoff, U.M. (Ed.) *Aspects of Oral Communication*. Berlin: Walter de Gruyter, 364-387.

Clark, S., Mangram, A., Ernest, D., Lebron, R. and Peralta, L. (2011). "Informed Consent: A Study of the Efficacy of Informed Consent and the Associated Role of Language Barriers". *Journal of Surgical Education* 68(2), 143-147.

Clyne, M. (1994). *Inter-cultural Communication at Work: Cultural Values in Discourse*. Cambridge: Cambridge University Press.

Conley, J.M. and O'Barr, W.M. (1990). *Rules versus Relationships: The Ethnography of Legal Discourse*. Chicago: University of Chicago Press.

Corbacho, C. (2011). "Programa medicación y multiculturalidad". *Universidad Autónoma de Madrid*. 15 junio 2012. http://www.uam.es/departamentos/filoyletras/antropologia_social/PMM/mediacion.html [Last accessed April 30th, 2014].

Cordella, M. (2004). *The Dynamic Consultation: A Discourse Analytical Study of Doctor–Patient Communication* (Vol. 128). Amsterdam/ Philadelphia: John Benjamins.

Corsellis, A. (2002). "Formación de los proveedores de servicios públicos para trabajar con intérpretes y traductores. Habilidades y competencias interculturales." In Valero-Garcés, C. (Ed.) *Traducción e Interpretación en los Servicios Públicos. Contextualización, Actualidad y Futuro*. Granada: Comares, 71-90.

—. (2009). *Public Service Interpreting. The First Steps.* Basingstoke, Hampshire: Palgrave Textbooks in Translating and Interpreting. http://us.macmillan.com/series/PalgraveTextbooksinTranslatingandInterpreting [Last accessed April 30th, 2014].

—. (2003). "Formación de los proveedores de servicios públicos para trabajar con intérpretes y traductores. Habilidades y competencias interculturales". *Traducción e Interpretación en los Servicios Públicos. Contextualización, Actualidad y Futuro*. Granada: Comares, 71-90.

—. (2006). "Making sense of reality". *Linguistica Antverpiensia, Special issue: Taking stock: research and methodology in community interpreting*, 341-352.

—. (2005). "Training interpreters to work in the Public Services". In Tennent, M. (Ed.) *Training for the New Millennium: Pedagogies for Translation and Interpreting*. Amsterdam/Philadelphia: John Benjamins, 153-173.

Cortes, L. and Camacho, M.M. (2005). *Unidades de Segmentación y Marcadores del Discurso*. Madrid: Arco/Libros.

Cost-effectiveness of Language Services Project Literature Review. (2008). http://www.imiaweb.org/uploads/pages/197.pdf [Last accessed April 30th, 2014].

Coupland, J. (2003). "Small talk: social functions". *Research on Language and Social Interaction*, 36, 1-6.

Coupland, J. (Ed.) (2000). *Small Talk*. London: Longman.

Coupland, J., Coupland, N. and Robinson, J.D. (1992). "'How Are You?': Negotiating phatic communion". *Language in Society,* 21, 207-230.

Coupland, N. and Ylänne-McEwen, V. (2000). "Talk about the weather: small talk, leisure talk and the travel industry". In Coupland, J. (Ed.) *Small Talk*. London: Longman, 163-182.

Coupland, N., Wiemann, J.M. and Giles, H.N. (1991). "Talk as 'problem' and communication as 'miscommunication': an integrative analysis". In Coupland, N., Giles, H.N. and Wiemann, J.M. (Eds.) *"Miscommunication" and Problematic Talk.* Newbury Park, London and New Delhi: Sage, 1-17.

Cushner, K. and Brislin, R.W. (1996). *Intercultural Interactions. A Practical Guide*. London: Sage.

Davidson, B. (2000). "The interpreter as institutional gatekeeper: the Social-linguistic role of interpreters in Spanish-English medical discourse". *Journal of Sociolinguistics* 4(3), 379-405.

Deber, R.B. (1994). "The patient-physician partnership: Decision making solving and the desire to participate". *Canadian Medical Association Journal*, 423-427.

Diaz-Cuellar, A., Ringer, H, and Schoeller-Diaz, D. (2013). "The Ulysses syndrome: migrants with chronic and multiple stress symptoms and the role of indigenous linguistically and culturally competent community health workers".
http://www.panelserver.net/laredatenea/documentos/alba.pdf
[Last accessed April 30th, 2014].

Díaz Martínez, F. (1999). "Asimetría profesional en la consulta de oncología: algunas constricciones conversacionales de la clínica". *Discurso y Sociedad*, 1(4), 35-68.

—. (2002). "La quimioterapia y sus efectos." In González Barón, M., Díaz Martínez, F. and Ordoñez Gallego, A. (Eds.) *La Relación Médico-Paciente. Una Visión Sociológica.* Barcelona: Ars Medica, 141-158.

Dodd, C. (1991). *Dynamics of intercultural communication*. Dubuque, IA: W.C. Brown Publishers.

Drew, P. and Sorjonen, M.L. (1997). "Institutional dialogue". In Van Dijk, T.A. (Ed.) *Discourse as Social Interaction,* London, Sage, 92-118.

Drew, P. & Heritage, J. (Eds.) (1992). *Talk at Work*. Cambridge: Cambridge University Press.
El Mundo. (2003). "Los médicos no entienden a los inmigrantes". *Elmundosalud.com*. http://www.elmundo.es/elmundosalud/2003/01/08/medicina/1042029513.html [Last accessed April 30th, 2014].
Ennis, S., Ríos-Vargas, M., and Albert N. (2011). "The Hispanic population: 2010". *2010 Census Briefs,* 2. Washington DC: United States Census Bureau.
Fairclough, N. (1995). *Critical Discourse Analysis.* London: Longman.
—. (1989). *Language and Power.* London: Longman.
—. (1995). *Critical Discourse Analysis.* London: Longman.
Fernando, S. (Ed.) (1995). *Mental Health in a Multi-ethnic Society.* London and New York: Routledge.
Ferraro, V. and Palmer K. (2005). "Differences between oral and written communication". *Speaking and arguing: the rhetoric of peace and war.* Mount Holyoke College: South Hadley, Massachusetts.
Finkelstein, D., Smith, M.K., Faden, R. (1993). "Informed consent and medical ethics". *Arch. Opthalmology,* 111(3), 324-326.
Fisher, S. and Todd, A.D. (Eds.) (1993). *The Social Organization of Doctor-Patient Communication* (2nd ed.). Norwood, NJ: Ablex.
Flores, G., Laws, M., Mayo, S., Zuckerman, B., Abreu M., Medina, L. and Hardt, E. (2003). "Errors in medical interpretation and their potential clinical consequences in pediatric encounters". *Pediatrics*, 111(1), 6.
Flores G., Abreu M., Barone CP., Bachur R. and Lin H. (2012). "Errors of medical interpretation and their potential clinical consequences: a comparison of professional versus ad hoc versus no interpreters". *Annals of Emergency Medicine,* 60(5): 545-53.
Fustel Fuentes, R. (2009-2010). "Análisis de las traducciones de materiales especializados en el ámbito sanitario en los servicios públicos". 51. Alcalá de Henares.
Galán Cortés, J.C. (1997). *El Consentimiento Informado del Usuario de los Servicios Sanitarios*. Madrid: Colex.
Galanti, G.A. (2004). *Caring for Patients from Different Cultures*. Philadelphia, PA: University of Pennsylvania Press.
García Valverde, M.D., Girela Molina, B. (2011). "Consentimiento informado: efectividad del mismo en la asistencia sanitaria a extranjeros". *Revista de Treball, Economía i Societat*, 60. Castellón: Comité Econòmic i Social de la Comunitat Valenciana.
Gargantilla, P. (2003). *Manual de Atención al Inmigrantes*. Madrid: Ergon.

Grubbs, V. et al. (2006). "Effect of Awareness of Language Law on language Access in the Health Care Setting". *Journal of General Internal Medicine*, 21(7), 683–688.

Grupo CRIT (2003). *Claves para la Comunicación Intercultural*. Castellón: Universitat Jaume I.

—. (2006). *Culturas Cara a Cara. Relatos y Actividades para la Comunicación Intercultural.* Madrid: Edinumen.

Gumperz, J. (1982). *Discourse Strategies*. Cambridge: Cambridge University Press.

Guerrero Zaplana, J. (2003). *Las Reclamaciones por la Defectuosa Asistencia Sanitaria: Doctrina, Jurisprudencia, Legislación y Formularios*. Valladolid: Lex Nova.

Gyomber, D., Lawrentschuk, N., Wong, P., Parker, F. and Bolton, D.M. (2010). "Improving informed consent for patients undergoing radical prostatectomy using multimedia techniques: a prospective randomized crossover study". *BJU International.*

Haffner, L. (2012). "Translation is not enough-interpreting in a medical setting". *The Western Journal of Medicine,* 157-257.

Hale, S. (2007). "Interdisciplinarity: Community Interpreting in the Medical Context". *Community Interpreting*. Hampshire: Palgrave Macmillan, 34-62.

Hamelink, C. (1998). "Human rights: the implementation gap". *Journal of International Communication*, 5, 54-74.

Healthcare Interpretation Network (2009). *National Standards Guide for Community Interpreteng Services*. HIN: Toronto, Canada.

Helman, C. (1990). *Culture, Health and Illness* 2. Oxford: Butterworth – Heinemann.

Heritage, J. (1997). "Conversation Analysis and Institutional Talk". In Silverman, D. (Ed.) *Qualitative Research: Theory, Method and Practice*. London: Sage, 161-182.

Herrero de Dios, A.; Reyes Martín, A.; García Areces, F. (2000). "Consentimiento Informado en un Área de Atención Primaria". *Atención Primaria*, 25(9) 61-9.

Heszen-Klemens, I. and Lapinkska, E. (1984). "Doctor-patient interaction, patients health behaviour and effects of treatment". *Social Science and Medicine* 19, 9-18.

Holmes, J. (2000). "Doing collegiality and keeping control at work: small talk in government departments". In Coupland, J. (Ed.). *Small Talk.* London: Longman, 34-61.

Hunt, L.M. and De Voogd, K. B. (2007). "Are good intentions good enough? Informed consent without trained interpreters". *J Gen Intern Med*, 22(5), 598-605.

Illiescu, C. (2006). "Sentido y sensibilidad en el papel del intérprete social en ámbito médico-sanitario en la Provincia de Alicante". *Actas del XXIV Congreso de AESLA celebrado en la UNED*. Madrid, 29-30 marzo de 2006.

International Medical Interpreters Association. *Standards of Practice*. Boston, MA: IMIA.

Jansà, J.M. (2008). "Políticas de salud pública e inmigración". In García Roca, J. and Lacomba, J. (Eds.) *Inmigración en la Sociedad Española: Una Radiografía Multidisciplinar.* Barcelona: Editorial Bellaterra, 865-874.

Kapland, S.H., Greenfield, S. and Ware, J.E. (1989). "Impact of the doctor-patient relationship on the outcomes of chronic disease". In Steward, M. and Roter, R. (Eds.) *Communicating with Medical Patients*. Newbury Park, CA: Sage, 28-235.

Kareen, J. and Littlewood, R. (1992). *Intercultural Therapy.* Oxford: Blackell Science.

Kaufert, J. and Putsch, R. (1997). "Communication through interpreters in healthcare: Ethical dilemmas arising from differences in class, culture, language and power". *The Journal of Clinical Ethics*, 8(1), 71-87.

Kelly, N. (2008). "Ethics and Standards". *Telephone Interpreting: A Comprehensive Guide to the Profession*. Victoria, CA: Trafford Publishing: 93-181.

King, P.E. (1991). "Communication, anxiety, and the management of postoperative pain". *Health Communication,* 3, 127-138.

Krewatch, A. (2012). *Two sides of the same coin: the perspective of English speaking patients and doctors in Madrid.* [Unpublished Master's Thesis]. Universidad de Alcalá, Madrid, Spain.

Krosin, M.T., Klitzman, R., Levin, B., Cheng, J. and Ranney, M.L. (2006). "Problems in comprehension of informed consent in rural and peri-urban Mali, West Africa". *Clinical Trials.*

Ku, L. and Flores, G. (2005). "Pay Now or Pay Later: Providing Interpreter Services in Health Care". *Health Affairs*, 24(2), 435-444.

Lázaro Gutiérrez, R. (2010). *Análisis del discurso institucional entre hablante nativo (HN) y hablante no nativo (HNN) en los servicios públicos*. [Unpublished doctoral dissertation]. Universidad de Alcalá, Madrid, Spain.

López Izquierdo, R.; Martín del Barco, O. and Álvarez, P. (2007). *Entrevista al Paciente Inmigrante.* Madrid: AMF, 3(5), 259-266.

López-Vélez, R. and Huerga, H. (2002). *Inmigración y salud. Aproximación desde Atención Primaria*. Madrid: PBM.

Llosada Gistau, J., Vallverdú Duch, I., Miró Orpinell, M., Pijem Serra, C. and Guarga Rojas, A. (2012). "Acceso y uso de los servicios sanitarios por parte de los pacientes inmigrantes: la voz de los profesionales". *Atención Primaria* 44(2): 82-88.

Long, A. (1983). "Linguistic and conversational adjustments to non-native speakers". *Studies in Second Language Acquisition* 5(2), 177-193.

Magalhães E. (2012). "Afraid? Who is afraid?". *The ATA Chronicles*. http://ewandromagalhaes.tempsite.ws/ARQUIVOS/PDF/ATA_CHRONICLE_MAR12.PDF [Last accessed April 30th, 2014].

Maslach, C. (1982). *Burnout, the cost of caring*. Englewood Cliffs, N.J.: Prentice-Hall.

Marshall, P.A., Adebamowo, C.A., Adeyemo, A.A., Ogundiran, T.O., Vekich, M., Strenski, T., Zhou, J., Prewitt, T.E., Cooper, R.S., Rotimi, C.N. (2006). "Voluntary participation and informed consent to international genetic research". *American Journal of Public Health.*

Martincano Gómez J. L. (2004). *Competencia Cultural en la Atención al Inmigrante. Talleres de Práctica Clínica en AP*. Madrid: SCM.

Martincano Gómez, J. L. (2003). *Manual de Medicina Transcultural*. Madrid: IMC.

Martincano Gómez, J. L. and García Campayo, J. (2004). *La Salud Mental en el Paciente Inmigrante.* Madrid: IMC.

Marticano Gómez, J. L., Rodríguez, V. M. G., Correales, R. G. and Campayo, J. G. (2004). *Los Problemas de Salud Mental en el Paciente Inmigrante*. Madrid: IMC.

Martín, M. and Phelan, M. (2009). "Interpreters and Cultural Mediators - Different but Completary Roles". http://www.academia.edu/250428/Interpreters_and_Cultural_Mediators_-_different_but_complementary_roles [Last accessed April 30th, 2014].

Maslach, C. and Leiter, M.P. (1997). *The Truth about Burnout: How Organizations cause Personal Stress and What to do about it*. (2nd ed.). San Francisco, CA: Jossey-Bass.

Maynard, D.W. (1991). "On the interactional and institutional bases of asymmetry in clinical discourse". *American Journal of Sociology*, 92, 448-95.

Meisel, A., Roth, L. (1981) "What we do and do not know about informed consent?". *Jama*, 246(21), 2473-2477.

Mesa, A. M. (2000). "The cultural interpreter: An appreciated professional. Results of a study on interpreting services: client, health care worker and interpreter points of view". In Roberts, R., Carr, S.E., Abraham D.

and Dufour, A. (Eds.) *The Critical Link 2: Interpreters in the Community*. Amsterdam/Philadelphia: John Benjamins, 67-79.

Metge, J. (1986). *In and Out of the Touch: Whakamaa in Cross-Cultural Context.* Wellington: Victoria University Press.

—. (1995). *New Growth from Old. Whaanau in the Modern World.* Wellington: Victoria University Press.

Metge, J. and Kinloch, P. (1978). *Talking Past Each Other: Problems of Cross-Cultural Communication*. Wellington: Victoria University Press/Price Milburn.

Mishler, E.G. (1994). "The struggle between the voice of medicine and the voice of the lifeworld". In Conrad, P. and Kern, R. (Eds.) *The Sociology of Health and Illness: Critical Perspectives*. New York: St. Martin's, 288-300.

Misra-Herbert, A., MD (2003). "Physician cultural competence: cross-cultural communication improves care". *Cleveland Clinic Journal of Medicine,* 70, 293- 296.

Musacchio, M. (2013). *El Impacto Psicológico de los Intérpretes en el Ámbito de la Salud Mental: El Caso del síndrome de Ulises.* [Unpublished Master's Thesis]. Universidad de Alcalá, Madrid, Spain.

Naranjo, C. (2009). "Cierra el servicio de mediación intercultural." *Madridiario.* 15 junio 2012. http://www.madridiario.es/2009/Enero/canal-social/124912/semsi-cierre-ayuntamiento-denuncia-psoe-zerolo-inmigracion-mediadores-dinamizadores-cear.html [Last accessed April 30th, 2014].

Narayanan, A. (2012). "Interpreters may help shorten hospital stays". *Chicago Tribune*. June 18th, 2012 http://articles.chicagotribune.com/2012-05-25/lifestyle/sns-rt-us-hospital-interpretersbre84o0z4-20120525_1_interpreters-patients-general-internal-medicine [Last accessed April 30th, 2014].

Navarro Moreno, S. (2012). *Interpretación en los Servicios Públicos. Impacto Psicológico y Emocional en el Intérprete. Análisis de Casos y Situaciones*. [Unpublished Master's Thesis]. Universidad de Alcalá, Madrid, Spain.

Olgierda, F. and Heidi, A. (2004). "Interpreting for the community". *Wake Forest University.* June 1st, 2012 http://lrc.wfu.edu/community_interpreting/pages/ad-hoc-interpreter.htm [Last accessed April 30th, 2014].

Olver, I.N., Whitford, H.S., Denson, L.A., Peterson M,J. and Olver, S.I. (2009). "Improving informed consent to chemotherapy: a randomized controlled trial of written information versus an interactive multimedia". *Patient Education and Counselling.*

Ong, L., De Haes, J., Hoos, A., and Lammes, F. (1995). "Doctor-patient communication: a review of the literature". *Social Science and Medicine*, 40(7), 903-918.

Ozolins, U. (1998). *Interpreting and Translating in Australia: Current Issues and International Comparisons.* Melbourne: Language Australia.

Pajares, M. (2007). *Inmigrantes del Este: Procesos Migratorios de los Rumanos*. Barcelona: Icaria.

Placencia, M.E and García, C. (2008). "Formas, usos y funciones del *habla de contacto* en español". Sección temática, *Oralia* 11.

Pöchhacker, F. and Kadric, M. (1999). "The hospital cleaner as healthcare interpreter: A case study". *The Translator*, 5(2), 161-178.

Poyatos, F. (1993). *Paralanguage: A Linguistic and Interdisciplinary Approach to Interactive Speech and Sounds.* Amsterdam / Philadelphia: John Benjamins.

—. (1976). *Beyond Words: Theory and Methodology of Nonverbal Communication.* New York, New York State English Council, (NYSEC Monographs, 15).

Raga Gimeno, F. (2005). "Médicos, marabouts y mediadores: Problemas de comunicación intercultural en la atención sanitaria a los inmigrantes de origen senegalés". In Valero-Garcés, C. (Ed.) *Traducción como Mediación Entre Lenguas y Culturas/ Translation as Mediation or How to Bridge Linguistic and Cultural Gaps.* Alcalá de Henares: Servicio de Publicaciones de la Universidad.

—. (2008). *Mediaciones Interculturales*. Valencia, Universitat de València: Lynx.

Ragan, S. L. (2000). "Sociable talk in women's health care contexts: two forms of non-medical talk". In Coupland, J. (Ed.) *Small Talk.* London: Longman, 268-287.

Rahman, I. Hirsch, J. and Shah, S. (2007). "Overcoming Language Barriers in the Criminal Justice System: Can Language Assistance TechnologyHelp?". http://www.empirejustice.org/archive/larc/newsitedesign/LEPTopics/LE/PoliceChiefArticle/Police%20Chief%20Magazine%20-%20View%20Article.htm [Last accessed: April 30th, 2014].

Riccardi, A., Marinuzzi, G., Zecchin, S. (2002). "Interpretation and stress". *Interpreting in the 21st Century.* Amsterdam/Philadelphia: John Benjamins, 93-105.

Roat, C. (2003). *How to choose and use a language agency: A guide for health and social service providers who wish to contract with language agencies.* Menlo Park, CA: The California Endowment.

—. (2006). *Certification of Health Care Interpreters in the United States: A Primer, a Status Report and Consideration for National Certification*. Menlo Park, CA: The California Endowment.

Salinas de Frías, C. (2008). "Problemas de salud de la población inmigrante y su relación con el sistema sanitario". In Salinas de Frías, A. (Ed.) *Inmigración e integración: aspectos sociales y legales*. Madrid: Ediciones Sequitur, 55-76.

Sánchez-Reyes, S. and Martín Casado, M. (2005). "Argumentos a favor de la implantación de un servicio de intérpretes en los hospitales". In Valero-Garcés, C. (Ed.) *Traducción como Mediación entre Lenguas y Culturas. Translation as Mediation or How to Bridge the Cultural Gap*. Alcalá de Henares: Servicio de Publicaciones de la Universidad de Alcalá.

Scollon, R. and Scollon, S. W. (1995). *Intercultural Communication*. Oxford: Blackwell.

Sarangi, S. and Roberts, C. (1999). *Talk, Work and Institutional Order*. Berlin: Mouton de Gruyter.

Schegloff, E. (1987). "The routine as achievement". *Human Studies*, 9, 111-151.

Schenker, Y., Wang, F., Selig, S.J., Ng, R. and Fernández, A. (2007). "The impact of language barriers on documentation of informed consent at a hospital with on-site interpreter services". *Gen Intern Med*, 22(Suppl 2), 294-9.

Secretaría General de Inmigración y Emigración. (2012). "Extranjeros residentes en España". *Ministerio de Empleo y Seguridad Social*. June 11th, 2012. http://extranjeros.empleo.gob.es/es/Estadisticas/ [Last accessed April 30th, 2014].

Sharf, B.F. (1988). "Teaching patients to speak up: Past end future trends". *Patients Education and Counselling*, 11, 95-108.

Simón Lorda P. and Concheiro L. (1993). "El Consentimiento Informado: Teoría y Práctica II". *Med Clin (Barc)*, 101(5), 174-182.

Simón Lorda P. and Concheiro-Carro L. (1993). "El Consentimiento Informado: Teoría y Práctica I". *Med Clin (Barc)*, 100(17), 659-663.

Simón Lorda P. and Barrio I. (1995). "El Consentimiento Informado y la Enfermería: Modelo Integral". *Jano*, 55-65.

Sim, A. (2012). "Spain enters new recession with worse to come, says central bank". *El País: in English*. June 13th, 2012 http://elpais.com/elpais/2012/04/23/inenglish/1335192339_820649.html [Last accessed April 30th, 2014].

Soriano, G. (2002). "La interpretación social en las instituciones hospitalarias de irlanda del norte". In Valero-Garcés, C. and Mancho,

G. (Eds.) *Traducción e Interpretación en los Servicios Públicos: Nuevas Necesidades para Nuevas Realidades*, 189-194.

Spencer-Oatey, H. (2008) (Ed.). "Introduction". In Spencer-Oatey. H. (Ed.) *Culturally Speaking: Culture, Communication and Politeness Theory* (2nd ed.) London: Continuum, 1-8.

Spencer-Oatey, H. and Franklin, P. (2009). *Intercultural Interaction. A Multidisciplinary Approach to Intercultural Communication*. Basingstoke: Palgrave/Macmillan.

Steward, R.L.Jr., Gold, W. R. and Mcdowell, T. (1995). "Discussing health related quality life in parental consultations". In Morris, G.H. and Chenail, R.J. (Eds.) *The Tasks in the Clinic: Explorations in the Analysis of Medical and Therapeutic Discourse*. Hillsdale, NJ: Erlbaum, 209-231.

Stone, D. (2007). *30 Days to Taming Your Stress*. Eufene, Oregon: Harvest House Publishers.

Taibi, M. (2006). "Estudio de la utilidad de traducciones para los servicios públicos". In García Blanco, P. and Martino, P. (Eds.) *Traducción y Multiculturalidad*. Universidad Complutense: Servicio de Publicaciones, 187-193.

Talero Martín, S. (1997). "La entrevista clínica". In Gil, V. F., Merino, J. and Quirce, F. (Eds.) *Manual de Metodología de Trabajo en Atención Primaria*. Alicante: Universidad de Alicante, 321-34.

Tannen, D. (1984). *Conversational style: Analyzing talk among friends.* Norwood, NJ: Ablex.

Tardón, L. (2009). "Los médicos españoles tienen pánico a hablar en inglés en los congresos". *El Mundo*. May 21st, 2012 http://www.elmundo.es/elmundosalud/2009/12/23/medicina/1261586856.html [Last accessed April 30th, 2014].

Tatum Krank, J., Shaykevich, Sh., Lipsitz, and S. and Soleymani, L. (2011). "Patient predictors of colposcopy comprehension of Consent among English- and Spanish-speaking Women". *Women's Health Issues*, 21(1), 80–85.

Thompson, T. L. (1994). "Interpersonal communication and health care". In Knapp, M. and Miller, G.R. (Eds.), *Handbook of Interpersonal Communication*. Thousands Oaks, CA: Sage, 696-725.

Terraza Núñez, R., Vargas Lorenzo, I., Rodríguez Arjona D., Lizana Alcazo, T. and Vázquez Navarrete, M. (2010). "Políticas sanitarias de ámbito estatal y autonómico para la población inmigrante en España". *Gaceta Sanitaria*, 24, 115-117.

Traber, M. (2008). "Communication is inscribed in human nature". *World Association for Christian Communication.* June 8th, 2012.

Tzanne, A. (2000). *Talking at Cross-Purposes,* Amsterdam/Philadelphia: John Benjamins.
UniversalDoctor. (2011). "Universal Doctor and Tools". http://www.universaldoctor.com/sect/en_GB/9002/Products.html [Last accessed April 30th, 2014].
U.S. Bureau of Labor Statistics. (2010). "Pharmacist" *U.S. Department of Labor*. May 31st, 2012.
Vaccarino J. (1978). "Consent, informed consent and the consent form". *New England Journal of Medicine*, 298(8), 455.
Valero-Garcés, C. and Dergam, A. (2001a). "¿Mediador social = mediador interlingüístico = Intérprete? Práctica, formación y reconocimiento del intérprete en los servicios sociales". *Sin Fronteras*, 3, 16-19.
Valero-Garcés, C. (2001b). "El mediador interlingüístico en los servicios públicos: ¿nuevos principios éticos para nuevas realidades?". *Últimas Corrientes Teóricas en los Estudios de Traducción*, 819-829. Salamanca: Servicio de Publicaciones de la Universidad.
—. (2001c). "Estudio para determinar el tipo y calidad de la comunicación lingüística con la población extranjera en los Centros de Salud." *OFRIM, Suplementos*, 117-132.
—. (2002a). "Modificaciones en la conversación institucional. Análisis de los turnos de habla en la entrevista clínica con pacientes inmigrantes". In Luque, G., Bueno, A. and Tejada, G. (eds.), *Las Lenguas en un Mundo Global,* Jaén: Servicio de Publicaciones de la Universidad, 29-38.
—. (2002b). "Análisis conversacional de las interacciones entre proveedores de servicios y usuarios inmigrantes en los centros de salud". *Oralia* 5, 265-296.
—. (2004). "Barreras lingüísticas en la comunicación intercultural. Datos y Acciones". *Ofrim* 11, 17-36.
Valero-Garcés, C. and Taibi, M. (2004). "Análisis de la interacción comunicativa en contextos institucionales entre proveedores de servicios, usuarios e intermediarios lingüísticos". *Oralia,* 7, 173-194.
Valero-Garcés, C. and Sales, D. (2005). "Translating for new multicultural realities: The complex nature of Translating as a socio-cultural practice". *JOSTRANS*, 7. http://www.jostrans.org/issue07/issue07_toc.php [Last accessed April 30th, 2014].
Valero-Garcés, C. (2005). "Doctor-patient consultations in dyadic and triadic exchanges". *Interpreting,* 7(2), 193-210.
—. (2006). "Emotional and Psychological Effects on Interpreters in Public Services. A Critical Factor to Bear in Mind".

http://www.translationdirectory.com/article537.htm [Last accessed April 30th, 2014].
—. (2008). "La conversación de contacto en contextos institucionales: la consulta médica". *Oralia*, 11, 107-131.
Valero-Garcés, C., and Martin, A. (Eds.). (2008). *Crossing Borders in Community Interpreting: Definitions and Dilemmas* (Vol. 76). Amsterdam/Philadelphia: John Benjamins.
Valero-Garcés, C. (2010). "Challenging communication in doctor / non-native patient encounters. Two perspectives, three types of interaction and some proposals". *The Journal of Specialised Translation*, 14, 230-242.
Watson, J. (1987). "Interpreter burnout". *Journal of Interpretation*, 4, 79–85.
West, C. (1990). "Not just doctor's orders". *Discourse & Society* 1(1), 85-112.
—. (1993). "'Ask me no questions': An Analysis of queries and replies in physician-patient dialogues". In D. Todd, A. D. and Fisher, S. (Eds.) *The Social Organization of Doctor – Patient Communication*, Norwood, NJ: Ablex, 127-157.
Williams, S.; Weinman J. and Dale, J. (1998). "Doctor-patient communication and patient satisfaction: a review". *Family Practice*, 15, 480-492.
Women's Clinic & Family Counseling Center. (2006-2010). "Routine gynecological exams." http://www.womens-clinic.org/routine_gynecological_exams.php [Last accessed April 30th, 2014].
Young, H. (2007). "Social norms". *Economics Series Working Papers,* University of Oxford, Department of Economics, 307, 3.

Useful Websites

American Translators Association (ATA): http://ata.net.org
Australian Government Department of Health and Ageing: http://www.health.gov.au/
Australian Society of Interpreters and Translators: http://www.ausit.org/
Chartered Institute of Linguists (IoL): http://www.iol.org.uk
Cross Cultural Health Care Program: http://www.xculture.org
Diversity RX: http://www.diversityrx.org
DPH Best Practice Recommendations for Hospital-Based Interpreter Services: http://www.mass.gov/dph/bhqm/2bestrapra.pdf
Graduate Medical School Admissions Test: http://www.gamsatuk.org/
Hands on Health South Carolina:

http://www.handsonhealth-sc.org/index.php
Harrison Online Access Medicine:
http://www.accessmedicine.com/public/learnmore_hol.aspx
Health Care Interpreter Network: http://www.hcin.org
Health Care For All: http://www.hcfama.org
Health and Literacy Compendium Home:
http://healthliteracy.worlded.org/docs/comp/Indexes/language.html
Institutos Nacionales de la Salud:
http://www.nlm.nih.gov/medlineplus/spanish
International Medical Interpreters Association:
http://www.imiaweb.org/
Medical monolingual dictionary: http://www.medterms.com/
Multilingual Health & Safety Resources:
http://www.lohp.org/hsresguide/library/doc/MULINGGUIDE3.pdf
Multilingual Health Education Net: http://www.multilingual-health-education.net/
National Council on Interpreting in Health Care: http://www.ncih.org
National Institutes ofHeatlh: http://www.nih.gov/
National LEP Advocacy Task Force: http://www.lwptaskforce.org
Office for Minority Health (including CLAS standards):
http://www.omhrc.gov/omhhome.htm
Refugee Health Information Network: http://www.rhin.org/Default.aspx
Transcultural Nursing Society: http://www.tcns.org

INDEX

Index of Authors

Subject Index